How to Really Prevent and Cure Heart Disease

ISBN: 978-1-68222-457-1

9 781682 224571

HOW TO REALLY PREVENT AND CURE HEART DISEASE

The Billion Dollar Cholesterol 'Scam' Exposed

Dr. Gottfried A. Lange, M.D.

— ABOUT THE AUTHOR —

Dr. Gottfried A. Lange graduated as a medical doctor in 1980 from Hamburg University in Germany. He specializes in the field of naturopathy and cellular nutrition, and the effects of chemical residues in the human body. Dr. Lange has researched the influences of drugs and environmental pollutants—such as heavy metals and pesticides—on human health and has consulted and published in the field of effective detoxification methods. He is a popular lecturer with consumers and health professionals on chemistry, toxicology, and the prevention and cures for common diseases including cardiovascular diseases and cancer.

— FOREWORD —

Without the important scientific work of Albert Szent-Györgyi, M.D., Ph.D., Roger J. Williams, Ph.D., G. C. Willis, M.D., Irwin Stone, Ph.D., Abram Hoffer, M.D., Ph.D., Linus Pauling, Ph.D., Matthias Rath, M.D., Alexandra Niedzwiecki, Ph.D., Walter Hartenbach, M.D., and Lothar Wendt, M.D., I could not have written this book. These scientists are the pioneers who worked to solve the puzzle of diseases affecting the blood vessels of the heart (cardiovascular diseases) and diseases affecting the blood vessels of other organs such as legs, kidneys and eyes (peripheral vascular diseases).

— CONTENTS —

—1—

Reducing Cholesterol Can Be Hazardous to Your Health

Are you more likely to die from heart disease if your blood cholesterol is high?

That would seem to be a reasonable assumption. Your doctor probably has told you so. You may have read about the dangers of high cholesterol in books, newspapers and magazines. Television ads touting cholesterol-lowering drugs certainly spread this idea.

However, statistics tell us that the number of people who die from a heart attack with a total cholesterol count over 300 *is not any greater than with cholesterol that is lower than 200.* [1, 2]*

In fact, of the patients admitted to hospitals for heart disease, 45 to 60 percent have what are considered as normal levels of cholesterol. [1, 3, 4]

What about the treatment for heart disease that is standard practice in modern medicine—the use of blood-fat and blood pressure-lowering drugs combined with intensive dietary cholesterol-lowering measures? Has this not reduced the incidence of heart disease? Again, statistics give us the true, unbiased picture: *Patients so treated have a 143 percent greater chance of dying from heart disease.* [5]

When we look further into this—again using scientific, objective methods—we find that the actual instances of death not caused by heart failure (such as cancer and diabetes) *more than double as total cholesterol levels drop below 160.* [1, 6]

From these statistics alone it becomes quite clear that forcing down cholesterol levels with drugs and drastic dietary measures is harmful to your health. Why is that?

---

*The figures in square brackets [ ] refer to the scientific documents listed at the end of this book.

Cholesterol is Vital for Your Health

Every single cell in your body contains a waxy, colorless substance called *cholesterol*.

Structural formula of cholesterol

Molecule of cholesterol

It is one of your most important biochemical building blocks. Cholesterol, in fact, is the foundation for a huge number of substances without which your body could not survive.

Cholesterol is especially important for the nervous system. It is a key molecule to build and maintain brain cells and all other nervous-system cells. Almost thirty percent of the body's cholesterol exists in the brain. It is not surprising that researchers have linked the onset of Alzheimer's disease to a lack of cholesterol. [1, 7]

Cholesterol is one of the key basic substances in the body for making many hormones and other vital substances. For example, the body makes vitamin D from cholesterol. Since vitamin D is needed for the absorption and metabolism of calcium, too little cholesterol can cause bones to become brittle and fragile (osteoporosis).

Sex hormones—both male and female—are made from cholesterol. A lack of cholesterol often means a reduced sex drive and reduced fertility. But sex hormones play a role not only in your desire for sex. They also regulate virility and fertility, and the formation of protein that builds strong muscles and flexible cartilage. Sleeping well also depends on normal levels of sex hormones. So a general weakness, lack of agility and tiredness can also be the result of too little cholesterol.

The total amount of cholesterol in your body is approximately 140 grams. This is a very large amount of a single substance and shows how important it is for your health. Of similar building-block substances, only calcium and phosphate exist in higher amounts.

What about the idea that high cholesterol causes heart attacks? Statistics tell otherwise. Twenty to twenty-five percent of those who are below the age of 50 and who die from a heart attack have a cholesterol level that is *lower than 180 mg/dl*. Conversely, many who have high levels of cholesterol do not show even the slightest narrowing of an artery (stenosis), according to a large, modern clinical study conducted at Frankfurt University in Germany. One of its researchers summarized the startling results: *"There has been no provable statistical correlation between the number and extent of arteriosclerotic stenoses of coronary arteries and total cholesterol levels."* [8, 9]

Over the last several decades, the death rate from heart disease in the U.S. has dropped by 60 percent. During the same period, the average cholesterol level decreased by only three percent. Such an insignificant decrease in the cholesterol level can hardly be the cause of that very large reduction in the number of people who die from heart disease. [10]

It is clear that another factor must be in play. Examining this further, we see that during this time period, there is a direct correlation between the decrease in the heart disease death rate and the *increase in vitamin C consumption.*

The more vitamin C a person takes, the lower are his chances of dying from heart disease. This relationship is the central subject of this book, something that I will examine in detail in following chapters.

Will heart attacks be unknown to future generations? The vitamin C connection is a discovery that certainly opens the door to the elimination of heart attacks. Why, then, has your doctor not told you about this? Why has cholesterol become the villain that we must fight to treat heart disease?

3

The Cholesterol "Scam"

"What If It's All Been a Big Fat Lie?" was the startling headline of a recent 8,000-word New York Times article by award-winning science writer Gary Taubes that met with astonishment and strong public interest. Exposing the massive cholesterol lowering drugs scheme initiated by the pharmaceutical companies, the article was later reprinted in the Wall Street Journal, the London Times and a number of other noteworthy newspapers. The article had such impact that it was then featured on CNN, ABC's Nightline, Larry King and the 20/20 television programs. Gary Taubes noted in his article: "If the members of the American medical establishment were to have a collective find-yourself-standing-naked-in-Times-Square-type nightmare, this might be it." [11]

The *National Heart, Lung and Blood Institute (NHLBI)* analyzed 19 scientific studies, involving 650,000 individuals and 70,000 deaths, about the role of cholesterol in heart disease. The researchers could find no evidence that cholesterol has any influence on the development of the progressive thickening and hardening of the walls of the arteries that we call arteriosclerosis—or any other forms of heart disease. In fact, the scientists noted that the higher the cholesterol level, the lower was the likelihood for the development of cancer or other forms of fatal disease. [12, 13]

You may ask, if all this is true, how can so many doctors be wrong? Why are these physicians continuing to prescribe cholesterol-lowering medication and recommend that you replace butter with margarine?

The answer to those questions is found in this statistic: The annual revenue to the pharmaceutical industry from cholesterol-lowering drugs is a staggering 40 billion dollars in the USA alone. [12]

Cholesterol is big business for Big Pharma.

The propaganda spread by these companies about cholesterol has been uncritically accepted by a majority of physicians. In their defense, doctors have been inundated since medical school with misleading information. And the risk of malpractice lawsuits, especially in the USA, for not using the "accepted" treatment for heart disease always hangs heavy over a doctor's head.

But the fact remains that a *very* large part of the profits of drug companies come from selling cholesterol-lowering drugs.

On the other hand, there exists much evidence of the *negative* effects from lowering cholesterol with drugs. Can it then be that the pharmaceutical industry hides and disguises these results for reasons of profit?

The original idea that cholesterol has a causative influence in the development of arteriosclerosis comes from an animal experiment almost one hundred years ago. A research team in Czarist Russia, headed by a man by the name of Alexander Ignatowski, reported in 1909 that changes "similar to arteriosclerosis" appeared in the aorta (the main blood vessel that carries blood from the heart to the rest of the body) in rabbits that were fed with eggs, milk and beef. [12]

It is interesting to note that eggs, milk and beef are not part of the natural diet of a rabbit. Nevertheless, the huge business that Big Pharma is making from cholesterol-lowering drugs has its genesis in that very old and very incomplete study.

The idea that cholesterol causes heart disease cannot be proven nor validated by any statistic. The effort to lower one's cholesterol is unlikely to prevent coronary heart disease and, in fact, does not reduce mortality. [14] Former astronaut, aerospace medical research scientist, flight surgeon and family doctor Dr. Duane Gravelin says in his book "Lipitor® – Thief of Memory – Statin Drugs and the Misguided War On Cholesterol": "Some would call this medical progress *but I can only call it failure!*" [15] Rather than focusing on the actual results, Big Pharma has put the spotlight on the very large number of people that were made to participate in the famous "cholesterol studies".

The statistics that were derived from these studies by the pharmaceutical industry were compiled using improper scientific criteria. Results that are supposed to prove that a high level of cholesterol causes heart disease are simply not there. Numerous prestigious scientists have evaluated this research and have found that it is "deceptive" and "misleading", that the results have been "manipulated" and "bent" and that the conclusions are "without scientific basis", "not useable", "superficial" and "absurd". [12, 16]

Here is a summary of the misinterpretations and the actual true results of these five most frequently quoted cholesterol studies:

The Scandinavian Simvastatin Survival Study (4S) (Oslo University, Norway, 1994): The results of this study involving 4,444 participants showed that elevated cholesterol levels have *no* influence on the development of arteriosclerosis or heart disease.

The Finnish Multifactorial Study (Helsinki Multifactorial Primary Prevention Trial, HMPPT, Helsinki University, Finland, 1985): This study, with 1,222 participants, usually heads the list of proof of the benefit of reducing cholesterol. The actual findings prove quite the opposite. They are an alarming warning against any attempt to lower cholesterol levels. The number of *heart attacks more than doubled* among the patients who were treated with antihypertensive and cholesterol-lowering drugs. The total death rate increased by more than 40 percent among those who received antihypertensive and cholesterol-lowering medications. [12, 13]

The Helsinki Heart Studies I and II (Helsinki University, Finland, 1987, 1993): The results of the Helsinki I study show no decrease of the number of deadly heart attacks, but a 40 percent increase of deadly side effects from lowering cholesterol. The follow-up Helsinki II study with the same cholesterol-lowering drug shows a 50 percent increase of heart attacks and a 50 percent increase of the total death rate. An after-analysis shows an increase of deaths from cancer by 43 percent.

The Framingham Heart Study (Harvard University Medical School, Boston, Massachusetts, ongoing study beginning in 1948): The purpose of this study (4500 participants) was to show the benefit of cholesterol-lowering drugs, something that could not be proven. And to cite the report: "For each mg/dl (milligram per deciliter) decrease in cholesterol there was an 11 percent increase in coronary and total mortality." Moreover, what also became quite clear from the study was that forcing down cholesterol levels led to a substantial increase of cancer deaths.

The Clofibrate Study: An alarming increase in cancer deaths among its 1000 participants led to an abandonment of this study. [12]

Professor Skrabanek at the University of Dublin in Ireland said of these studies: *"Nothing in the field of medicine has ever proven so completely the lack of success of those efforts to make cholesterol responsible for coronary heart disease."* And he added: *"The pharmaceutical industry tried to bend the statistics until they fit their pipe-dreams."* [12, 17]

Rather than proving that cholesterol is the cause of heart disease, the five cholesterol studies have shown us that [12]:

1. **Cholesterol has *no* influence on the development of arteriosclerosis or heart disease.**

2. ***High* cholesterol levels are associated with a *high* life expectancy and *low* incidence of cancer.**

3. ***Lowering* cholesterol levels is associated with numerous deaths and the *increased* incidence of cancer.**

— 4 —

Cholesterol Drugs and Disease

Any lowering of cholesterol is not only useless; it is hazardous to your health. And, it is often deadly. [12]

In January, 1996, with the headline *"Cancerogenicity of Lipid-Lowering Drugs"*, the prestigious Journal of the American Medical Association (JAMA) announced to the medical community the correlation between cholesterol-lowering drugs and cancer.

Dr. Thomas Newman and Dr. Stephen Hulley of the University of San Francisco, California, revealed that *all* cholesterol-lowering drugs currently taken by millions of people worldwide are potentially cancer causing. Two classes of such drugs, the so-called fibrates and statins, are particularly carcinogenic. The medical profession was warned against the use of these medicines. [18, 19]

Professor Walli at University Hospital Munich-Grosshadern in Germany, discovered that *every* person who suffers from cancer has a very low cholesterol level due to an insufficient supply of cholesterol to the cells. For example, a total cholesterol count of below 160 triples the risk for a women dying from lung cancer. [20, 21]

How can a lack of cholesterol cause cancer?

The human body consists of approximately 50 trillion cells. The cells are the body's biochemical factories, the basic units of physical life. Cholesterol is essential for building and maintaining the exterior cell wall as well as every partition inside the cell that makes up its complex inner structure.

Each biochemical reaction in the "cell factory" is tied to a specific *location* on the inner cell structure. Cholesterol is an indispensable construction material that makes this structure whole and intact. Without cholesterol, these membranes cannot exist. When you reduce the amount of cholesterol, you then weaken vital cell structures. The cells begin to deteriorate. They become more prone to carcinogenic mutation. And cancer-fighting cells of the immune system become less effective. [12, 22, 23]

Cholesterol-lowering drugs (statins) cause a deficiency in coenzyme Q10. Coenzyme Q10 is a vital "cell fuel" substance. In order to cope with its heavy workload the heart needs sufficient supplies of coenzyme Q10. A healthy heart has the highest coenzyme Q10 contents of any organ. To date, there are 15 published trials on statin-induced Q10 depletion in humans. A lack of Q10 reduces the concentration of the coenzyme in the heart and leads to eventual heart failure. But this is not all. A general coenzyme Q10 deficiency causes a deterioration of outer and inner cell walls, malfunction of energy production, malfunction of immune functions, increased risk of Alzheimer's disease, cardiovascular disease, cancer and Parkinson's disease. [7, 24, 25, 26]

Also Dr. Peter Langsjoen, well-known cardiologist and researcher at the University of Texas Health Center, has observed that statins can even cause what they are supposed to cure. He reports a "frightening increase in heart failure" in connection with statin usage. [25, 27]

A substantial number of cases of impotence associated with cholesterol-lowering statin drug usage has been reported [27A, 27B].

If you are pregnant or considering becoming pregnant, there is one group of medications to be added to the long list of drugs you should not take because they can harm your baby: the cholesterol-lowering statin drugs. Researchers at the U.S. National Institutes of Health found that the use of statins during the first trimester of pregnancy is associated with severe central nervous system defects and limb deformities in the fetus. These findings, published in a research letter in the April 8, 2004, issue of the New England Journal of Medicine, reported that 20 of 52 babies exposed to statins in the womb were born with malformations. [28]

Statin drugs are also bad for your mental health. They have caused depression and increased the risk of suicide when the cholesterol level drops below 160. [29, 30, 31, 32] A significant association between low or lowered cholesterol levels and behavioral violence is found across many types of scientific studies. [33, 34] Too little cholesterol also appears to be related to the onset of Alzheimer's disease. [7]

The German magazine, *Stern,* reported in the August 16, 2001, issue that pharmaceutical companies work hard to motivate and encourage a doctor to become what is known in Big Pharma jargon as a "good prescriber" of cholesterol-lowering statin drugs. These companies know that a patient who is put on a statin drug will take it for the rest of his or her life. The magazine gave examples how the Bayer pharmaceutical company had offered cash, travel on the Orient Express and other incentives for doctors who met their statin prescription quotas.

Professor Borgers of the Berlin Social Science Research Center— the largest research institute of its kind in Europe—comments in his book *"Cholesterol - the Failure of a Dogma"* that the propaganda by Big Pharma falsifying the role of cholesterol has penetrated family medicine and mislead a whole society that cholesterol is the villain that must be fought at all cost. [35]

Let's take a closer look at this intriguing substance called cholesterol.

— 5 —

An Evaluation of Cholesterol

Cholesterol is the starting substance for the biosynthesis of many of our most important hormones. The term *hormone* refers to a biochemical substance that controls cell and tissue function. One of these is **cortisol**, our most important stress hormone. Its primary functions are:

- To activate glucose and fatty acids, the sources of energy for each cell, and

- to activate the minerals potassium and sodium, which regulate the entirety of our physical and cerebral performance.

Dr. Hartenbach, university researcher and teacher, specialist in vascular surgery, with decades of research on nutritional diseases, cancer, and vascular diseases, found that moderate stress, such as from athletic competition, causes a two- to four-fold increase in cortisol production. More severe stress—such as that from surgery, an accident or top-level athletic competition of longer duration—can boost cortisol levels by a factor of ten. [12, 16]

When cortisol levels go up, the liver increases its cholesterol production. Incidentally, the liver produces 85 percent of the body's cholesterol—only 15 percent comes from food.

Cortisol in the body keeps allergies in check. It improves blood clotting by increasing the number of blood platelets and therefore helps to stop bleeding. Cortisol stabilizes the heart and blood circulation, and regulates blood pressure. It prevents uncontrolled cell growth and division, including that of cancerous cells.

Without cortisol, your body could not perform physically and this would have a direct and negative impact on mental processes as well. Without cortisol there would be no physical life. Since cholesterol is the starting material for cortisol, you can see how dangerous it can be to reduce cholesterol with cholesterol-lowering drugs.

Cholesterol is also the starting substance for the biosynthesis of the male and female **sex hormones**. These hormones are, of course, responsible for sexual function. But they also control the formation of muscles and bones—and they regulate your sleep.

Dr. Max Otto Bruker, renowned physician and one of the world's leading researchers on nutritional medicine, writes in his book "Cholesterol—the Vital Substance": *"If the popular press would tomorrow broadcast that without sufficient cholesterol, there would be no capacity of sex or reproduction, the cholesterol problem would at once be resolved. The reputation of butter would be restored and the whole scam would be over. The need for cholesterol for a good sex life cannot be overemphasized."* [36]

The main functions of sex hormones include:

- Male potency;
- Female fertility;
- Building up of muscle protein (sex hormones are also known as anabolics);
- Controlling the incorporation of stabilizing protein and calcium into the skeletal system, which in turn prevents osteoporosis;
- Regulation of sleep.

Cholesterol is the starting substance for the biosynthesis of the hormone **aldosterone**, which regulates your body's entire mineral metabolism.

It is also the starting compound for the body to manufacture the **bile acids** that regulate fat digestion and bowel movement.

Cholesterol is needed to make **vitamin D**, which in turn is essential for building and maintaining stable bones and joints. Sufficient levels of vitamin D appear to lower an individual's risk of developing certain cancers—including colon, breast, and ovarian cancer—by up to 50 percent, according to cancer prevention specialists at the Moores Cancer Center at the University of California, San Diego (UCSD) Medical Center. [37]

Last but not least, cholesterol is the **primary building block** for the walls of the trillions of cells in the body. These cells carry out the functions of your organs and keep the body alive.

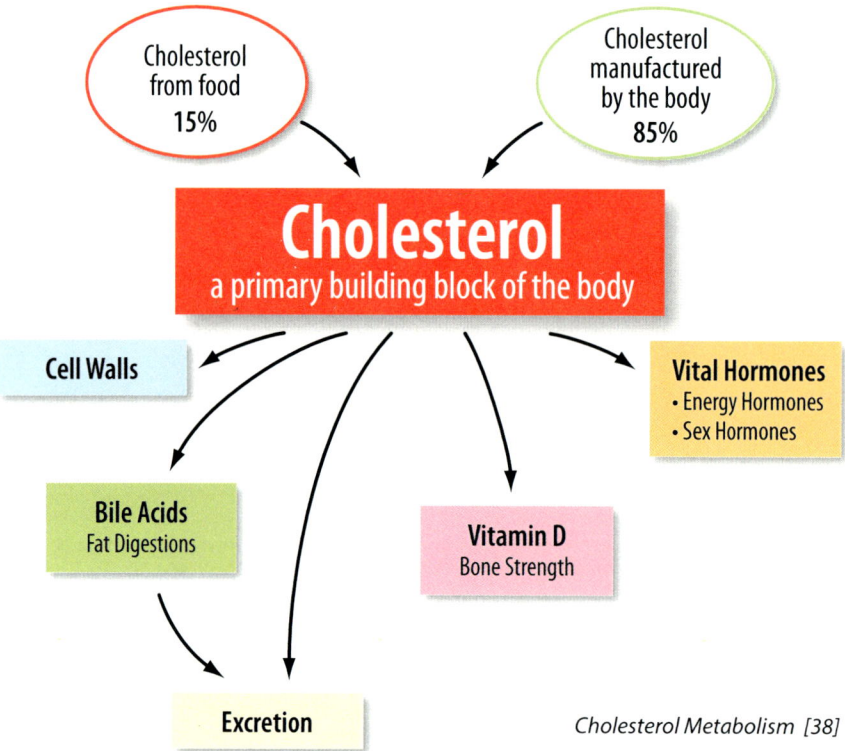

Cholesterol Metabolism [38]

Cholesterol is not a dangerous, villainous substance but rather one of the most essential and valuable building blocks of your body.

'Good' cholesterol and 'bad' cholesterol is a marketing myth which has taken hold and has generated billions of dollars in cholesterol lowering drugs and products. The truth is that there are two different biochemical cholesterol transport compounds: LDL

(Low Density Lipoprotein) and HDL (High Density Lipoprotein). These two compounds have different functions. LDL transports cholesterol from the liver where it is manufactured to the cells of the body. HDL transports cholesterol to the liver. The myth of 'good' and 'bad' cholesterol stems from misconceptions that cholesterol builds up in the arterial walls because LDL transports cholesterol to the cells. While this is not true, how this *actually* works is explained in detail later in this book.

It is the false claim that every adult with a cholesterol level above 200 mg/dl (milligrams per deciliter) is to be considered ill and therefore in need of medical treatment that has further supported the billion dollar drug and cholesterol lowering industry. If this false claim were true, it would mean that practically the entire adult population of the world would be labeled ill and in need of treatment. And, while this may be a 'reassuring' business premise for drug company stockholders and investors, it totally neglects the needs, health and well-being of the consumers.

The *average* total cholesterol level worldwide for adults is 250 mg/dl (80 to 90 percent of the adult population). Values up to 350 mg/dl are not unusual. They are, in fact, still normal, point to a considerable vitality and should actually be evaluated positively. [12]

There is not only evidence that people with high cholesterol live the longest, but also that high cholesterol even protects against infections and arteriosclerosis [38A].

Cholesterol levels of 400 mg/dl to 1000 mg/dl and above point to a metabolic disorder of the mitochondria (the energy generation plants of the body) or to a hereditary hypercholesterolemia. This disease is caused by a lack of receptor (cholesterol receiving) molecules on the surface of the cells. As a result the absorption of cholesterol into the cells is seriously decreased—and, with that, the vital cholesterol supply for the sealing of the cell walls and for the mitochondria (the energy production plants in the cells). This situation causes an ever-increasing blood cholesterol level. Over the years this leads to cholesterol deposits in all of the organs and eventually the blood vessel walls; however, these deposits have nothing in common with arteriosclerosis (the common human arterial disease), and have in fact quite a different appearance. The continuous lack of cholesterol in all cells leads to premature exhaustion of cell division and to consequent multiple cancerous growths.

The following chart shows the average and upper cholesterol levels for the population in the USA. The chart also points out from which values on upwards **non-medicated** treatments of a possible metabolic disorder could be indicated.

Cholesterol Blood Levels (mg/dl = milligrams per deciliter) [12]

Age	Average Level	Upper Limit	Treatment Required
10 - 19	175 mg/dl	230 mg/dl	approx. from 300 mg/dl
25 - 29	198 mg/dl	270 mg/dl	approx. from 350 mg/dl
40 - 59	50 mg/dl	350 mg/dl	approx. from 400 mg/dl
65 - 85	slightly decreasing	330 mg/dl	approx. from 400 mg/dl

It is important to note that when measuring cholesterol levels, one needs to keep in mind that they are subject to considerable fluctuations. Physical and mental stresses increase the liver's production of cholesterol in order to provide the body with what it actually needs to meet and deal with the additional challenges. This is not unusual and should be taken into account when one attempts to measure cholesterol levels. One may have to measure the cholesterol several times before one gets a clear picture of what the cholesterol level actually is on average.

The main point here is: Cholesterol is one of the key building substances for all of the body's cells and for many vital hormones. It enables optimum cellular structure and function. Cholesterol regulates and stabilizes physical life in all areas of the body. It is the substance that guarantees the longevity and the orderly division of cells, thus protecting the body from cancerous degeneration. [12]

— 6 —

How to Safely Lower Cholesterol Levels
When Really Needed

There are several effective ways to lower out-of-range cholesterol without the use of pharmaceutical drugs.

First among these is vitamin C. This vitamin is necessary for the body to produce bile acids from cholesterol. Vitamin C enables and increases such synthesis, thereby lowering cholesterol levels naturally. Numerous scientific studies show that vitamin C also lowers high blood fat levels and also protects these lipids against harmful oxidation. [12, 18, 39 - 44]

Niacin in dosages of 1.5 to 3 grams per day lowers lipoprotein(a)—the main risk factor for arteriosclerosis and heart disease (see chapter 10 for details)—by 10 to 35 percent. One can start with as low a dose as 100 mg taken three times each day after meals and gradually increase it. Niacin reduces cholesterol and LDL by 10 to 20 percent and triglycerides by 30 to 70 percent, increases blood-clot dissolving activity in blood vessels, increases HDL by 20 to 35 percent and slightly lowers blood. [24, 45, 46]

Many other studies prove that niacin lowers excessive blood lipid levels. [46 - 50]

Abram Hoffer, M.D., Ph.D., researcher and editor of the international "Journal of Orthomolecular Medicine", said in a 1997 interview: "Pharmaceutical companies are very annoyed with niacin because their products have to compete with it. Some of their cholesterol-lowering drugs cost up to $150 a month, while niacin costs only about $10."

Vitamin B5 (pantothenic acid) lowers cholesterol and tri-glycerides and elevates HDL cholesterol. [51, 52]

Vitamin E increases HDL cholesterol and protects blood fats against oxidation, which would otherwise convert these lipids into aggressive particles that damage the walls of blood vessels. [53, 54]

L-Carnitine optimizes cellular fat metabolism and lowers high triglyceride levels. [18, 55, 56]

One to six grams of cinnamon per day reduces blood sugar levels by 18 to 29 percent. It also lowers triglycerides by 23 to 30 percent, LDL cholesterol by 7 to 27 percent and total cholesterol by 12 to 26 percent. [57]

Numerous studies show that pectin has favorable effects on lipids. Pectin is classified as a soluble fiber; it is found in most plants, but is primarily concentrated in citrus fruit (oranges, lemons, grapefruit) and apples. [58 - 72] So it is wise to eat more cereals, vegetables and other fiber-rich foods to "flush out" excessive cholesterol from the body naturally. [18]

Lets now turn to an examination of the real factors that put you at risk for the development of cardiovascular disease and how to effectively and naturally prevent this illness.

The Heart Disease Epidemic

Every year, over the world, an estimated 17 million people die of cardiovascular diseases, particularly from heart attacks and strokes. [73]

In the U.S. alone, 2000 people die daily from heart attacks.

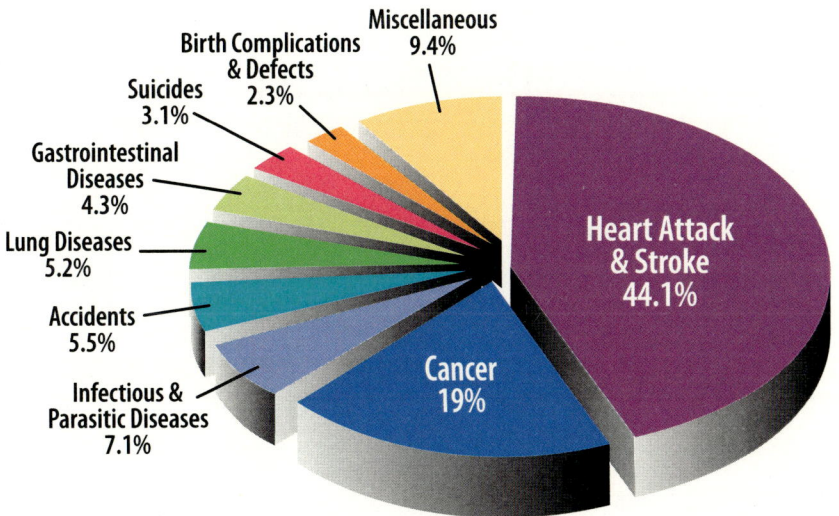

World Health Report
Causes of Death

63 out of 100 people die from Cardiovascular Disease or Cancer

Every second man and woman in the industrialized world suffers and eventually dies from the consequences of arteriosclerotic plaques—the repair deposits in your arteries that lead to thickened artery walls and narrowed inner artery diameters. The further this repair process progresses, the less blood can flow through the arteries.

Healthy Artery

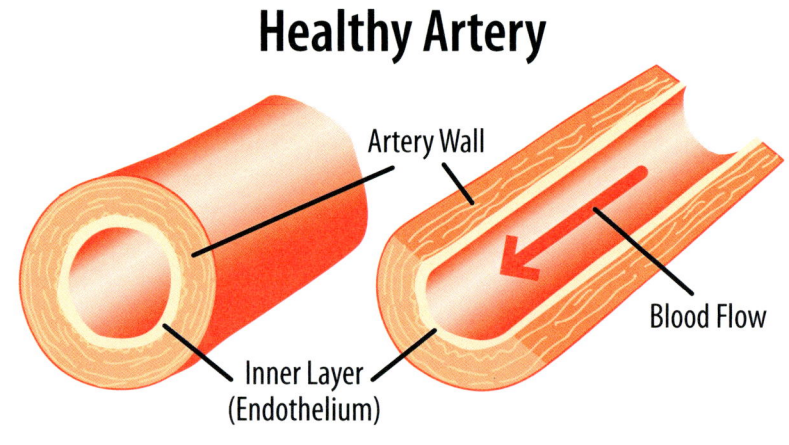

Artery Wall

Blood Flow

Inner Layer
(Endothelium)

Diseased Artery
Reduced Blood Flow

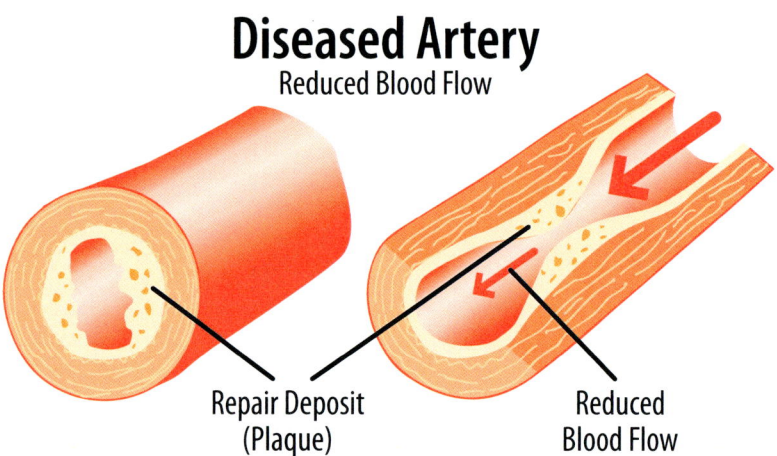

Repair Deposit
(Plaque)

Reduced
Blood Flow

Then if a blood clot blocks one or more of your coronary arteries, it leads to a heart attack. If a blood clot blocks the arteries that supply blood to the brain, the result is a stroke.

Diseased Artery
Blocked Blood Flow

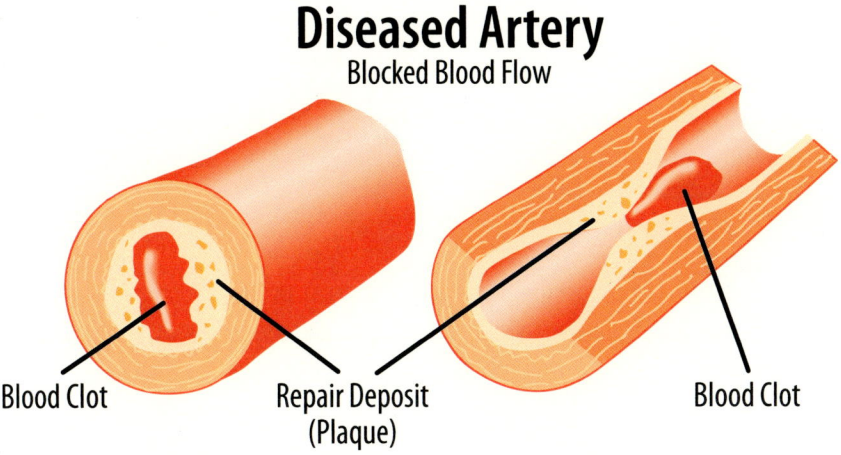

Blood Clot

Repair Deposit
(Plaque)

Blood Clot

Cardiovascular disease has become an epidemic because, until recently, we have not understood the true nature of arteriosclerosis and coronary heart disease. [18]

This "cardiovascular epidemic" is one of the largest economic burdens for America and other countries. The direct and indirect costs associated with this disease amount to trillions of dollars worldwide each year. [18]

But recent research has shown that cardiovascular diseases are not genuine diseases at all, but rather *the result of long-term deficiencies of vital natural biochemical substances in the cells of the walls of blood vessels.* [74, 75]

Because of this new scientific breakthrough, it is now possible to effectively and economically treat cardiovascular disease—and also to prevent it. [75, 76]

Let's now examine this in more detail. To understand this, we first have to look at how our cells work.

How Cells Work

Cells are the smallest autonomous living units in the body. They are the body's biochemical assembly plants, power stations and biochemical waste elimination plants.

The diameter of a cell is between 10 and 50 micrometers (millionth of meters). There are roughly 50 trillions of cells in the human body.

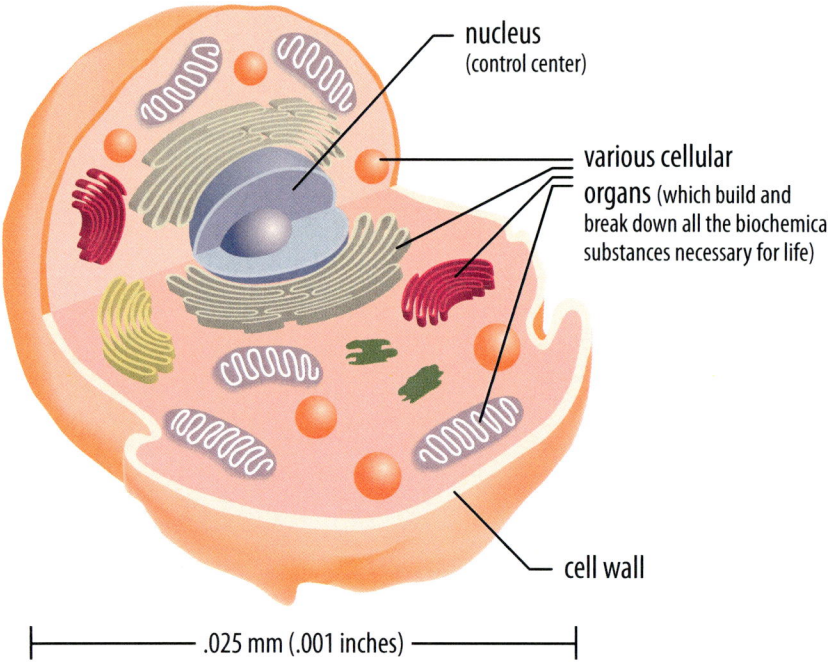

nucleus (control center)

various cellular organs (which build and break down all the biochemical substances necessary for life)

cell wall

.025 mm (.001 inches)

These cells assemble and dismantle thousands of different substances using biochemical tools called *enzymes*.

Most of these enzymes consist of two parts, an *apo-enzyme*, a kind of 'handle' consisting of protein, and a *co-enzyme*, which can be seen as an 'inset' that completes the enzyme and makes it into a usable tool called *holo-enzyme*.

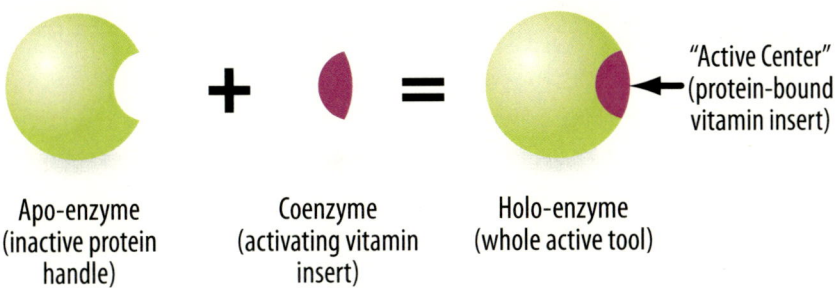

"Active Center"
(protein-bound
vitamin insert)

Apo-enzyme
(inactive protein
handle)

Coenzyme
(activating vitamin
insert)

Holo-enzyme
(whole active tool)

The co-enzyme represents the "active center" of the enzyme. It is the part that is directly involved in the biochemical reaction. [77]

Somewhat simplified, this is comparable to a screwdriver (holo-enzyme) that consists of a handle (apo-enzyme) and an insert bit (co-enzyme). The bit makes it possible to perform certain tasks. Without a bit the screwdriver is useless.

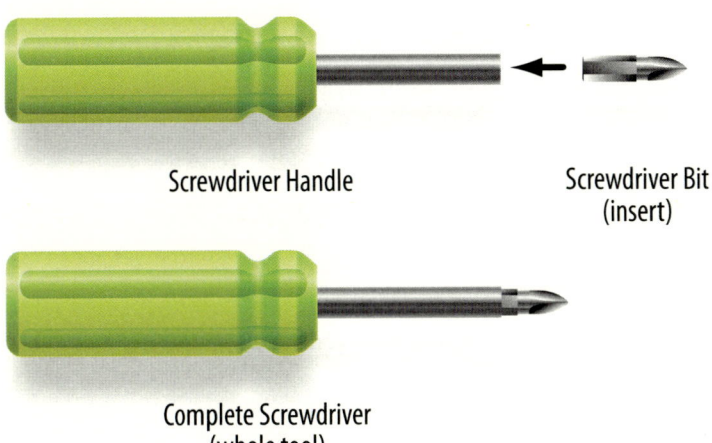

Screwdriver Handle

Screwdriver Bit
(insert)

Complete Screwdriver
(whole tool)

Most co-enzymes cannot be manufactured (synthesized) by cells in the body and thus have to be ingested with the daily food or as supplements. A well-known word for most of these co-enzymes is *vitamins*. The vitamins are the 'insert bits' for the enzymes that enable the enzymes to function.

If there is a lack of such biochemical tool substances—vitamins—a cell cannot work at an optimum level, and this eventually leads to chronic diseases like cardiovascular diseases, diabetes, or cancer.

Approximately 100,000 biochemical reactions take place in each cell every second through the activity of co-enzymes. It is obvious that these cells must receive a regular supply of these co-enzymes—vitamins—otherwise the cells and your health begin to deteriorate.

Because there is a continuous 'wear' of these 'screwdriver bits'—coenzymes or vitamins—there must be a continuous re-supply of 'replacement parts'. If this does not take place, there is a progressive shutdown of the human cellular factory, leading to fatal disease and eventual death.

Deficiencies in vitamins and trace elements are very common today for several reasons:

- There are not enough vitamins and trace elements in the food we eat due to modern agricultural and industrial food processing methods.

- Our environment, including the food we eat, has become chemically polluted.

Normally, plants absorb approximately 60 different minerals and trace elements from the soil. However, common chemical fertilizers usually contain only nitrogen, phosphorus and potassium. This leads to a lack of minerals and trace elements, and it causes a reduced biosynthesis of many vitamins in the plant. In addition, extensive industrial food processing destroys or leaches out many such vitamins and trace elements.

This table of the average vitamin content in selected foods in 1985 and 1996 illustrates this:

Vitamin / Food (100 g)	1985	1996
Beta-carotene	4.7 mg	1 mg
Vitamin B6	0.33 mg	0.022 mg
Vitamin C	5 mg	1 mg

Over four million distinct chemical compounds have been reported in the scientific literature since 1965. Each week 6,000 new compounds are added to the list. Of these, as many as 100,000 are currently in commercial production.

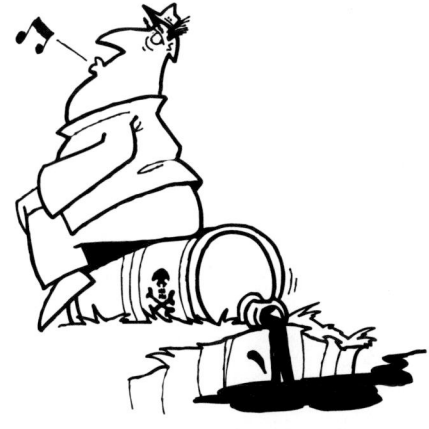

Human exposure to these chemicals is both direct and indirect. More than 3,500 chemicals are deliberately added to food and over 700 have been identified in drinking water. These, together with pharmaceutical and recreational drugs, cause a considerable chemical stress in people. In addition, because man is at the top of the food chain, the chemicals accumulate more in the bodies of humans (bio-magnification). The average American has between 400 and 800 chemicals in their body. [78]

Chemical food additives and other pollutants make the vitamin deficiencies inside and outside of cells worse: More vitamins are used up in the body to cope with "scavenging" aggressive pollutants. This reduces the amount of vitamins—the 'screwdriver bits'—available in the body for other vital biochemical tasks.

There is today a widespread lack of such vital biochemical 'tool' substances as vitamin C, vitamin E, magnesium, and others, causing

General Nutritional Situation

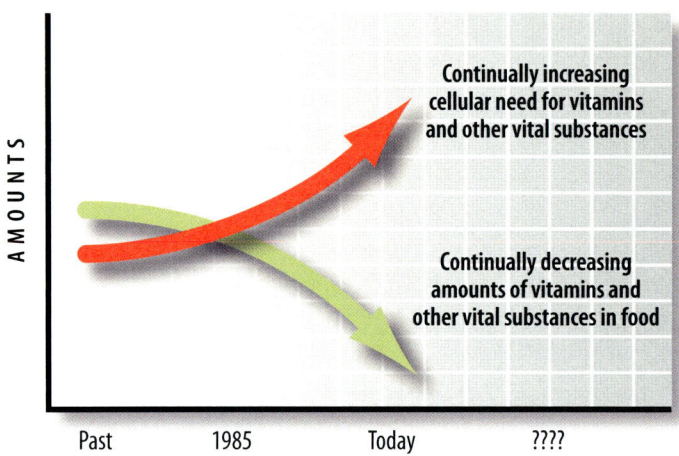

extensive cellular deficiencies. Compounding this is the cellular stress caused by the ever-increasing discharge of environmental pollutants using up vitamins and other essential 'tool' substances at a progressive rate. With this development still continuing, the result can be disastrous for your health, unless you take proactive steps to correct it.

Because of these external stress factors on cells—the progressive lack of vitamins and other vital substances in food and, in addition, an increased need of them for capturing and neutralizing chemical pollutants—good nutrition alone is no longer sufficient to meet the body's requirements for these vital 'tool' substances. The old adage "just eat more fruit and vegetables" is no longer a solution.

Summarizing the results of the latest research, two-time Nobel laureate Linus Pauling has this advice: *"The optimum daily amounts of vitamins are far larger than the amounts that can be obtained in food, even by selecting foods for their high vitamin content. The only way to obtain the amounts of vitamins that put you in the best of health is to take vitamin supplements."* [79]

By the way, checking blood levels of vitamins is not a reliable method to establish your cellular vitamin status. There can be a lack of vitamins in the cells that does not show up in your blood. [80]

Where Heart Disease Begins

The wall of an artery has three layers.

In the *inner* layer, the structural elements are arranged primarily in a longitudinal direction. This is because the blood flow puts a stress on the wall chiefly in the direction of the bloodstream.

Arterial Wall

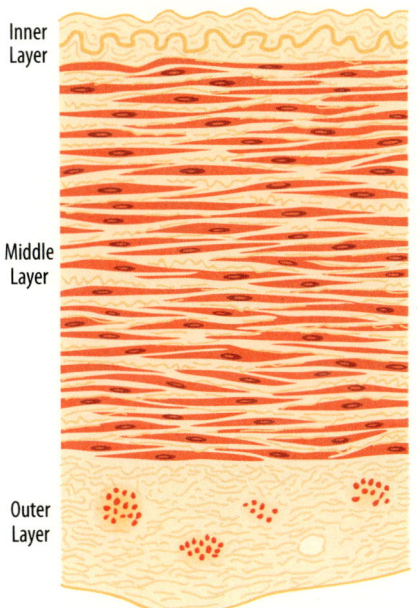

Inner Layer

Middle Layer

Outer Layer

The *middle* layer is adapted to pulsation and dilation and runs predominantly in a circular pattern.

The *outer* layer connects up with the surrounding connective tissue and has to be able to flex because of the pulsations. Its component parts are arranged like a concertina barrier of a predominantly longitudinal mesh. This structure is comparable to the nylon mesh built into the plastic of a garden hose to strengthen and stabilize it.

The inner layer (the "endothelium") consists of cells and two types of fine fibers: collagenic and elastic.

The collagenic fibers are made of a protein substance called collagen, which forms not only blood vessels but also skin, bones, teeth, cartilage, eyes, heart—in fact essentially all parts of the body. Without collagen the body would be a formless heap of cells. Collagen exists as strong white fibers, stronger than steel wire of the same weight (so strong that a strand with a diameter of 1/32nd of an inch can hold a weight of 15 to 20 pounds), and as yellow elastic networks (elastin). These fibers and networks form the connective tissues that hold our bodies together. [79]

The middle layer consists of a thick layer of tight, spirally-arranged muscle cells. Among these is a small amount of elastic and collagenic connective tissue.

The outer layer consists mainly of longitudinally running collagen fibers, with some smooth muscle cells. The elastic fibers in the blood-vessel wall are connected to each other and with the elastic fibers of the surrounding tissue, forming a three-dimensional lattice. [81]

The **key characteristics of healthy arterial walls** are **stability** and **elasticity** provided by the connective tissue (consisting of collagen and elastin fibers).

In order to build and to maintain **strong and elastic arterial walls**, the smooth muscle cells of the arteries need to produce high-grade collagen and elastin fibers.

To be able to produce high-grade collagen and elastin fibers, the cells need first and foremost the biochemical tool that we know as vitamin C. **Without sufficient supply of vitamin C, the cells are unable to produce healthy and strong collagen and elastin fibers. Consequently, the walls of the blood vessels begin to deteriorate.**

This is the true cause of cardiovascular disease.

And this is the crucial point: Your dog and your cat make their own vitamin C. So do most other animals; however, **the human body cannot manufacture its own vitamin C**.

Interesting and illuminating research, published in several well-known scientific journals from 1976 to 1994, has been carried out by Dr. Nishikimi and fellow researchers at the Department of Biomedical Chemistry, Nagoya University, Japan. It is probable that some millions of years ago, due to a genetic mutation, our ancestors lost the ability to make vitamin C from blood sugar (glucose). [74, 75, 83 - 89]

The human body now depends utterly on vitamin C from what we eat—but there is by far not enough vitamin C in what we eat today.

Premature cardiovascular disease (CVD) is essentially unknown in all animal species that produce their own high amounts of vitamin C.

In contrast, in man, unable to produce his own vitamin C, cardiovascular disease has become the number one disease. [87]

Most mammals synthesize vitamin C, usually in the range of 30 to 300 mg per kilo (13 to 130 mg per pound) of body weight. [74] Converting this to a man with the average weight of 150 pounds gives us a necessary daily vitamin C intake of approximately 2,000 to 20,000 mg per day. This range has been further confirmed by scientific research. [87]

For patients who are at high risk, a daily vitamin C intake in the range of 10,000 to 20,000 mg, or more, is recommended. This corresponds to the amount of vitamin C our distant ancestors synthesized in their body before we lost this ability. [74, 75, 83, 84, 87]

The best-known and most obvious consequence of vitamin C depletion in the cells is scurvy. Scurvy develops because of an extreme depletion of vitamin C resulting in blood vessels becoming fragile and brittle, leading to massive internal bleeding throughout the body and to death [83, 90]

Today, the condition of total depletion of vitamin C leading to scurvy with its complete loss of the integrity and stability of vascular walls and associated internal bleeding is very rare. This is because it takes very little vitamin C to camouflage it. Arteriosclerosis, which leads to cardiovascular disease, is really a hidden, insidiously slow progressing form of scurvy.

Such an insufficient supply of vitamin C in the cells of the vascular wall that leads to the deterioration of the vascular wall is very common today. By the age of 25, one out of every two people has begun to develop arteriosclerosis, without displaying any particular symptoms (yet).

The Villain—Lipoprotein(a)

When there is a continuous deficiency of vitamin C in cells that cover the inside of blood vessels (endothelium cells), the shape of these cells changes and large gaps begin to form between them. [75, 91]

This makes the inner layer of the blood-vessel wall (endothelium) more porous and permeable, thus opening the door to the infiltration of repair particles such as lipoproteins. A lipoprotein is a spherical particle consisting of a globule of fat (lipid) molecules surrounded by a protein shell.

The most sticky of these lipoproteins is called Lipoprotein(a)— usually abbreviated Lp(a). [92]   The (a) in its name stands for "adhesive". Lp(a) consists of two protein shells surrounding a fat (lipid) core that closely resembles LDL (low-density lipoprotein, which has been incorrectly named as a marker for the risk of heart disease). [74, 93, 94] Lp(a) is the most specific repair particle among all lipoproteins. It is effective in tissue repair processes such as wound healing. [87]

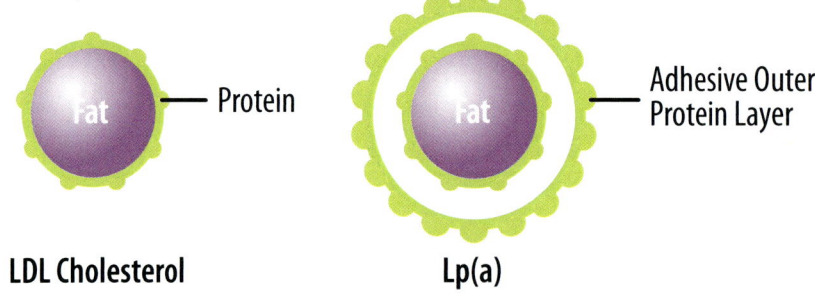

LDL Cholesterol   Lp(a)

A chronic vitamin C deficiency also causes the connective tissue that is the main building material of the blood vessel walls, to become loose and fragile. Thus, the stability and elasticity of the blood vessels deteriorate. [75]

To compensate for this, the body increases the blood levels of blood-vessel-constricting and blood-clotting substances, among them a potent protein called fibrinogen (preliminary form) and subsequently fibrin (final form) that is involved in forming blood clots. As the wall of a blood vessel becomes more porous, more fibrinogen is deposited in the blood vessel wall in order to prevent bleeding. [75]

Simultaneously, the liver increases its production of Lp(a), thereby also increasing the amount of Lp(a) in the blood. The Lp(a) particle is the ideal repair molecule. Lp(a) enters the loosened arterial wall and accumulates there in order to repair it. [95] However, with chronic insufficient dietary vitamin C intake, this defense mechanism overshoots.

More and more Lp(a) enters the weakened arterial wall and accumulates there in order to repair the gaps. [95] Lp(a) can bind to the cells coating the inside of the blood vessels (endothelium cells). [96, 97, 98] Lp(a) binds to fibrin in the blood vessel wall. [96, 99, 100] One of the attributes of Lp(a) is that it prevents fibrin and thus clots from being dissolved. [101]

The essentials of cardiovascular disease: The fiber framework stabilizing the blood vessel walls, becomes loose and fragile due to a chronic vitamin C deficiency. As a defense action, fibrin and Lp(a) plug the holes. Smooth muscle cells grow into the fragile areas. Some calcium is deposited to help stabilize the arterial wall. But this repair becomes an overrepair, especially in areas of high blood pressure such as in the heart arteries. The affected artery becomes more and more narrow until a small blood clot is enough to shut down the artery. That is cardiovascular disease. In the following paragraphs this is explained in more detail. [75, 76, 87]

In this way, a chronic vitamin C deficiency, through the deposition of fibrin and Lp(a) in the blood vessel walls as a defense mechanism, leads to a general thickening of all blood vessel walls throughout the circulatory system. But this does not necessarily lead to the development of arteriosclerotic plaques (swellings within the artery walls which lead to narrowed arteries and thus a decreased blood flow). If, however, a more intense blood flow in certain locations—

such as in the heart muscle—increases the stress on the blood vessel wall and reveals the underlying impairment, more repair particles are deposited in such a location and plaques develop as a countermeasure. [75]

This explains why human arteriosclerosis develops mainly at sites where there is a strong blood flow and thus an increased stress on the arterial wall: around the heart where the arteries are bent or squeezed 100,000 times every 24 hours (coronary arteries), and at the neck (cervical arteries) and brain (cerebral arteries) where the arteries branch. This is where the systolic blood pressure—the peak in pressure in the arteries caused by a contraction of the heart—is particularly high.

It also explains why the primary manifestations of human cardiovascular disease are heart attack and stroke, and also why high blood pressure increases the risk of cardiovascular disease. An increased blood pressure throughout the circulatory system extensively reveals the underlying weakness of the arterial walls. [75]

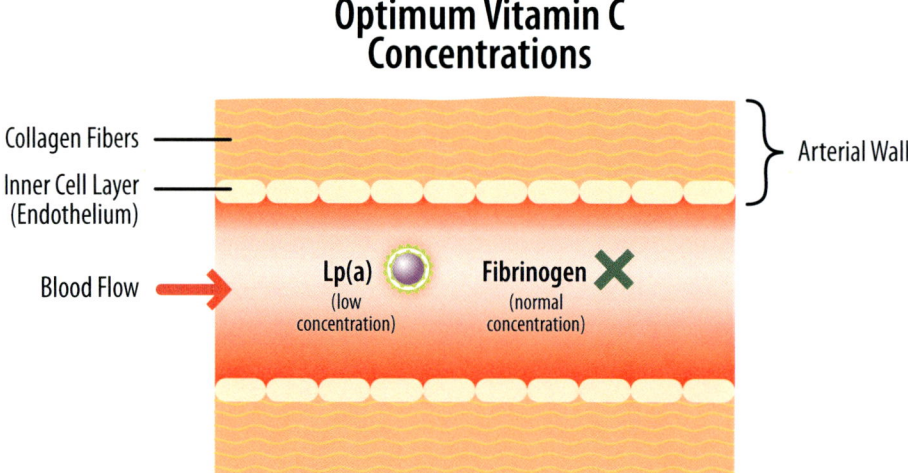

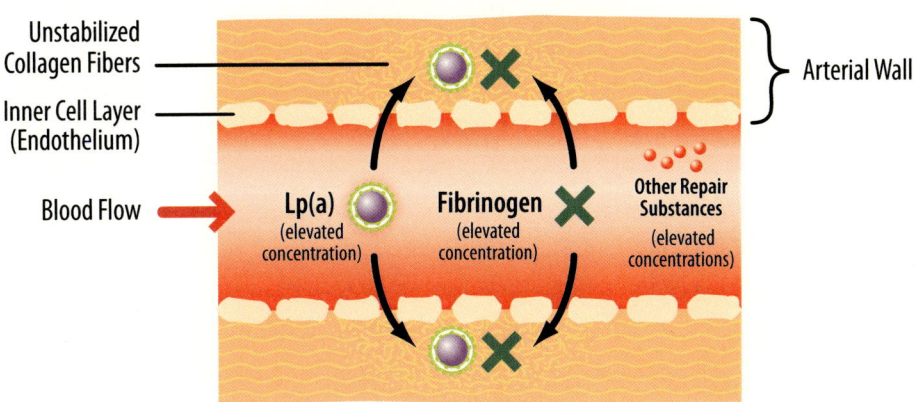

Vitamin C Deficiency
Normal Blood Flow Intensity

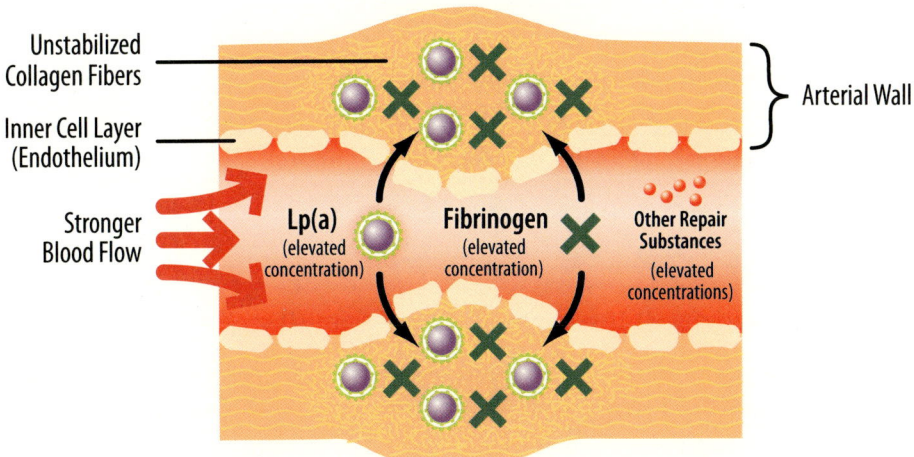

Vitamin C Deficiency
Sites of Stronger Blood Flow

From: Rath M, Pauling L: Solution of the puzzle of human cardiovascular disease: Its primary cause is vitamin C deficiency, leading to the deposition of lipoprotein(a) and fibrinogen/fibrin in the vascular wall. J Orthomol Med 1991; 6: 125-134. [75]

Numerous studies have now confirmed that **Lp(a), not LDL cholesterol, is the primary lipoprotein responsible for initiating the development of arteriosclerosis**.

Comprehensive studies directed by Dr. Ulrike Beisiegel, dean of research at the Hamburg University Hospital and chairperson of the European Atherosclerosis Society, directly addressed this issue. These studies assessed the role of Lp(a) in human blood vessel walls and found that Lp(a), not LDL cholesterol, accumulates selectively in the blood vessel walls of cardiovascular disease patients. Moreover, the researchers found that accumulation of Lp(a) in the arterial walls closely correlates to the development of arteriosclerotic plaques in both the human aorta (main blood vessel) and the coronary arteries (the vessels that supply blood to the heart muscle). [75, 95, 96, 100]

Most importantly, hundreds of tissue samples from human coronary arteries and the aorta (the main blood vessel) show that deposition of LDL alone in the artery walls occurs very rarely. [100] The reason that the initiation and formation of arteriosclerotic plaques was earlier attributed to LDL appears to be due to inadequate analytical methods; earlier investigators failed to differentiate between LDL and Lp(a). [95]

Further evidence that cholesterol is not the cause of arteriosclerosis, heart attack, stroke, and other cardiovascular diseases, is the fact that at most only *one percent of the content of arteriosclerotic plaques is cholesterol* [12].

The French magazine, *Nouvel Observateur*, in a major article on cholesterol, posed this question: "Is this cursed molecule responsible for our whole misery?" And then promptly provided the answer: "Nothing else has as little scientific backup as this."

Prior to 1989, the year when Dr. Linus Pauling and Dr. Matthias Rath uncovered the reason for heart disease, few studies existed on Lp(a). Since then, the research into Lp(a) science has exploded. There are now more than 1700 studies and articles about Lp(a) in the MedLine medical database alone.

The research has confirmed that the degree to which Lp(a) is deposited in the arterial wall directly correlates to the extent of plaque development in both the human aorta and the coronary arteries. [100] Furthermore, the studies show that Lp(a) and vitamin C blood levels are inversely correlated: The lower the vitamin C level, the higher the Lp(a) level; the higher the vitamin C level, the lower the Lp(a) level. [74, 102]

A striking relationship between Lp(a) and vitamin C, discovered by Dr. Matthias Rath in 1987, is that only species that have lost the ability to synthesize vitamin C—humans, other primates, and the guinea pig—have detectable amounts of Lp(a) in their blood. Lp(a) and vitamin C blood levels are inversely correlated to each other (please see preceding paragraph) in wound healing, arteriosclerosis, cancer, diabetes, and other pathological conditions, in these species. [74]

Connections between Lipoprotein(a) and Vitamin C [10]

Lipoprotein(a)	Vitamin C
is found *only* in humans, other primates and guinea pigs in considerable amounts	is a vitamin *only* for humans, other primates and guinea pigs
seals arteries in the heart and arteries in other organs by deposition	strengthens arteries by synthesis of collagen and elastin; lack of it leads to porous blood vessels
is an antioxidant (prevents oxidation)	is an antioxidant (prevents oxidation)
strong increase leads to arteriosclerosis	lack of it leads to arteriosclerosis

There is **no** correlation between Lp(a) levels and cholesterol blood levels. Among CHD (coronary heart disease) patients with normal blood fat levels, the only risk factor for coronary heart disease is elevated Lp(a). [95] Lp(a) above 30 mg/dl (milligrams per deciliter) doubles the risk of coronary heart disease, and if in addition LDL is elevated the CHD risk is increased by a factor of 5. [103]

Blood levels of the main risk factor Lp(a) [10]

Blood Level (mg/dl)	Risk
below 20*	small
20 to 40	moderate
above 40	very high

* From 0 to 10 the risk is higher than from 10 to 20, possibly the vascular wall "sealing" at very low levels is relatively poor.

There is now strong clinical and experimental evidence that the repair molecule Lp(a) is a much more important risk factor than total cholesterol or LDL-cholesterol for arteriosclerosis, coronary heart disease [104, 104A], stroke [105, 106], as well as restenosis of vein grafts after coronary bypass surgery [107]. High Lp(a) blood levels increase the risk for arteriosclerosis and cardiovascular disease five-fold. Any high Lp(a) blood level constitutes a ten-times higher risk than a correspondingly high total cholesterol or LDL-cholesterol level. [10, 108] More alarmingly, a study published in "Circulation", a journal of the American Heart Association, even shows that cholesterol-lowering drugs (statins) *increase* Lp(a) blood levels. [109]

There is no correlation between Lp(a) and the other "blood fat levels" (such as total cholesterol, LDL-cholesterol, HDL-cholesterol, and triglycerides). This means that a person with a "normal" cholesterol level can have a high Lp(a) level and thus a high risk for arteriosclerosis, heart attack, and stroke. [10, 110]

This explains the occurrence of arteriosclerosis in individuals who have a normal body weight, normal cholesterol levels, have neither high blood pressure nor diabetes, who do not smoke and who exercise. Despite conventional theories that such individuals should not develop any heart condition, they can develop coronary heart disease and suffer heart attacks. A high Lp(a) blood level is why. [10, 110]

—11—

Coming to the Rescue: Vitamin C

Weight loss regimens, cholesterol-lowering diets, or "modern" cholesterol-lowering drugs have no influence on Lp(a). Only the following natural substances lower Lp(a) levels:

- Vitamin C [39, 74, 75, 111, 112, 113, 114]
- Niacin [47, 115, 116]
- Coenzyme Q10 [117]
- Omega 3 fatty acids [118]
- Acetylcysteine [119]

A deficiency in vitamin C triggers all the risk factors leading to arteriosclerosis and blood clotting. [75] **Vitamin C supplementation**, on the other hand, reduces these risk factors and has the following beneficial effects:

- Vitamin C increases *prostacyclin*, a hormone that widens the blood vessels and inhibits the clotting of blood platelets. [75, 120]

- Vitamin C increases *EDRF (endothelium-derived relaxing factor)*. EDRF is a natural biochemical messenger which is manufactured by the cells that cover the inside of the walls of our blood vessels (endothelium cells). It relaxes the muscle cells in these arterial walls, thus widening the arteries and lowering blood pressure. [75]

- Vitamin C decreases *thromboxane*, a hormone that promotes clotting of blood platelets. [75]

"Vitamin C is essential for the building of collagen, the most abundant protein built in our bodies and the major component of connective tissue. This connective tissue has structural and supportive functions which are indispensable to heart tissues, to blood vessels - in fact, to all tissues. Collagen is not only the most abundant protein in our bodies, it also occurs in larger amounts than all other proteins put together. It cannot be built without vitamin C. No heart or blood vessel or other organ could possibly perform its functions without collagen. No heart or blood vessel can be maintained in healthy condition without vitamin C." — Dr. Roger J. Williams, renowned researcher and professor at Texas University [121]

- Vitamin C decreases *fibrinogen*, a precursor to fibrin. [75, 87] Fibrinogen is one of the components forming arteriosclerotic plaques. Moreover, fibrinogen is involved in forming blood clots.

- Vitamin C decreases *Lp(a)*, which is the most important risk factor for the development of arteriosclerosis, heart attack, and stroke. [122]

- Vitamin C prevents *Lp(a)* deposition in the walls of blood vessels. [122]

- Vitamin C reduces the affinity of the blood-vessel walls for binding with *Lp(a)*. [75]

- Men who take high-doses of vitamin C have between two and three times less *calcification* in their arteries. [123]

- Vitamin C preserves the integrity of the blood-vessel walls and therefore prevents the formation of *arteriosclerotic plaques*. [122]

- Vitamin C decreases the lipoproteins *LDL* and *VLDL*. [124]

- Vitamin C decreases *cholesterol* and *triglycerides*. [87]

- Vitamin C increases the lipoprotein *HDL*. [125]

- Vitamin C protects triglyceride-rich lipoproteins such as VLDL from being oxidized to substances that damage the walls of blood vessels [126], increases the production of *lipases*—enzymes (biochemical tools) that break down *triglycerides* and thereby lower triglyceride levels [40, 87], quenches harmful substances including destructive oxygen particles from tobacco smoke, and regenerates vitamin E that also quenches such harmful substances. In these ways, vitamin C protects the peripheral blood vessels—such as blood vessels in the legs, kidneys, eyes etc.—from oxidative damage. Such damage would otherwise lead to arteriosclerosis and circulatory problems in these areas (peripheral vascular disease). [75]

- Incidentally, besides the subject of cardiovascular disease, a study conducted by Dr. Brody, researcher and professor at the University of Paisley, Scotland, concluded that 3000 mg of oral vitamin C daily even increases sexual potency. [127]

Vitamin C provides all these benefits at the same time. It would be quite impossible for any pharmaceutical product to be more effective than vitamin C—a substance that has been developed and improved by nature over billions of years.

Premature arteriosclerosis is essentially unknown in most animals, whereas millions of humans, with chronic vitamin C deficiency, die of arteriosclerosis and related diseases, such as heart attack and stroke, each year. [75]

The prevention of heart disease and stroke normally requires about three grams of vitamin C per day. Much higher dosages are needed to remove existing arteriosclerotic plaques. Vitamin C is best taken throughout the day to ensure that there is no deficiency. The smaller each single dose, the higher is the percentage that is absorbed. [128]

MORE SCIENTIFIC STUDIES AND THEIR RESULTS

A high vitamin C intake protects against heart disease. It has long been known that when you eat plenty of fruits and vegetables—foods that are rich in vitamin C—heart disease occurs more rarely. A study with nearly 12,000 Americans conducted by Dr. Enstrom, an internationally recognized researcher at the School of Public Health, University of California, Los Angeles, demonstrated that a daily vitamin C intake of 300 to 600 mg reduces heart disease by approximately 40 percent and increases life expectancy by about 6 years. [129]

Reduction in the death rate, compared to the "normal" death rate in the United States, in persons taking supplementary regular daily vitamin C in doses ranging from 300 to 600 mg vitamin C per day. [129]

	Total Death Rate	Death Rate Heart Disease	Death Rate Cancer
All Persons	- 23%	- 34%	- 18%
Men	- 35%	- 42%	- 22%
Women	- 10%	- 25%	- 15%

A high vitamin C blood level protects against heart disease and stroke. Several studies have confirmed this. [113, 130, 131, 132]

A study conducted by Dr. Joel A. Simon, University of California, San Francisco, found that for every 500 microgram (millionth of gram) increase in vitamin C blood concentration an 11 percent reduction in coronary heart disease and stroke could be anticipated [132A].

In another study conducted by Dr. Gey, professor and researcher at Bern University, Switzerland, **beta-carotene** was administered to physicians who had arteriosclerosis, as a protective substance. This resulted in a **reduction of heart attacks and death rate** by 40 to 50 percent. [113]

Increase in the risk of heart disease and stroke in persons with low blood levels of vitamin C and beta-carotene [113]

Antioxidant	Risk for heart disease	Risk for stroke
Low vitamin C	+25%	+ 28%
Low beta-carotene	+53%	+107%
Low vitamin C and low beta-carotene	+96%	+300%

Influence of increased vitamin C or vitamin E intake on death rate through heart disease [*129, **133, ***134]

Number of persons examined	Increased vitamin C intake	Increased vitamin E intake	Reduction of death rate from heart disease (by percent)
4479 Men*	> 300 mg		42%
6879 Women*	> 300 mg		25%
39910 Men**		> 75 mg	36%
87245 Women***		> 75 mg	34%

Note: The symbol > means "more than".

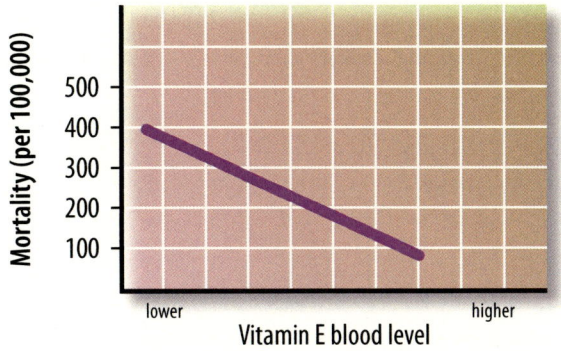

Inverse relation between vitamin E blood levels and death rate from ischemic* heart disease in different European countries [135]

(*ischemic: relating to or affected by ischemia; ischemia: a shortfall in blood supply)

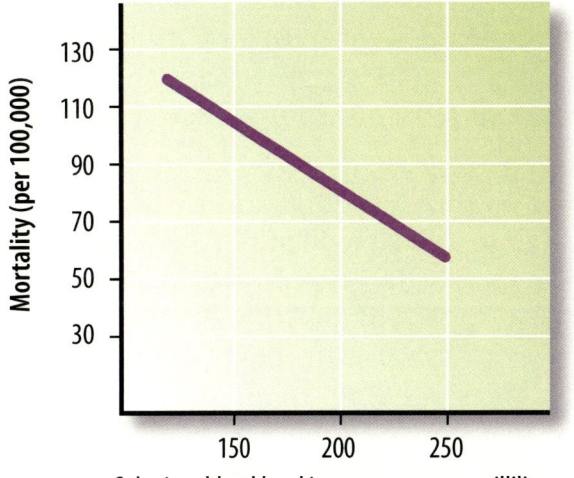

Selenium blood level and mortality from cardio-vascular disease [136, 137]

In a study sponsored by the American Heart Association, Dr. B. Sokoloff, M.D., Ph.D., of the Washington University School of Medicine, showed that two to three grams of vitamin C per day could lower triglyceride blood levels by an average 50 to 70 percent. Vitamin C increases the production of lipases (enzymes able to break down triglycerides) and thereby lowers triglyceride levels. Vitamin C increases the synthesis of these lipases by up to 100 percent. [18, 40]

Niacin (nicotinic acid, nicotinamide, vitamin B3) lowers Lp(a) levels by about 30 percent, apparently by reducing the rate at which Lp(a) is synthesized. Niacin was earlier used to lower lipid levels. When niacin was used, the death rate from heart disease dropped as well as the total death rate. [47, 115, 116]

Smoking is one of the main risk factors for the development of arteriosclerosis. Contrary to the popular view, it is not the nicotine that causes this. Nor does smoking increase cholesterol levels. But what is hazardous are the many aggressive substances that are in cigarette smoke. **Smokers have lower vitamin C blood levels** because vitamin C is used up to neutralize these aggressive chemicals. One cigarette uses up about 25 mg of vitamin C. The RDA (Recommended Daily Allowance, the daily amount that the Food and Drug Administration recommends) for vitamin C in the U.S. is only 60 mg. If a person smokes only two cigarettes per day that absurdly low amount of vitamin C is used up—just for the cigarettes.

Homocysteine is a harmful substance formed by the decomposition of the amino-acid methionine. Elevated homo-cysteine levels lead to an increased risk for damage to blood-vessel walls and their subsequent arteriosclerotic repair. Homocysteine levels increase when you are deficient in the vitamins B6, B12, and folic acid. You can therefore easily control this by taking a B-complex supplement that contains sufficient amounts of these vitamins (as well as of vitamin B2). [138] Also acetylcysteine lowers elevated homocysteine levels. [139, 140, 141]

How to Prevent and Reverse Heart Disease

"The enjoyment of the highest attainable standard of health is one of the fundamental rights of every human being without regard to race, religion, political belief and economic or social condition." [Excerpt from the World Health Organization's Constitution]

"Nature,
to be commanded,
must be obeyed."

— Sir Francis Bacon
British philosopher, essayist, statesman, 1561-1626

Dr. Albert Szent-Györgyi, who in 1927 first isolated vitamin C from cabbage and oranges and from the adrenal glands of oxen, and W. M. Haworth, an English biochemist and a pioneer in research on carbohydrates, who discovered its structural formula, called the substance ascorbic acid, meaning the acidic sub-stance that prevents and cures scurvy. [79] Dr. Györgyi received a Nobel Prize for his discovery in 1937.

Sixty-four years ago, vitamin C deficiency was first recognized as a prominent risk factor in cardiovascular disease. [142] Fifty-one years ago vitamin C was shown in Xray examinations of blood vessels to reduce arteriosclerotic plaques in man. [143, 144] There is no rational explanation why these early observations of the therapeutic value of vitamin C were ignored and why they have not become common knowledge among the medical profession. [75]

In 1967, the American chemist Dr. Irwin Stone found that almost everyone suffers from the genetic disease hypoascorbemia (deficiency of vitamin C in the blood), and that the vitamin C dose required for prevention of disease is 50 times the officially recommended daily dose of 60 mg per day for adults. [145]

Dr. Albert Szent-Györgyi, who first isolated ascorbic acid, wrote to Dr. Linus Pauling in April 1970: *"As to ascorbic acid, right from the beginning, I felt that the medical profession misled the public. If you don't take ascorbic acid with your food you get scurvy, so the medical profession said that if you don't get scurvy you are all right. I think that is a very grave error. Scurvy is not the first sign of the deficiency but a premortal* (occurring before death) *syndrome* (a set of physical conditions that show you have a particular disease or medical problem), *and for full health you need much more, very much more."* [79]

Dr. Linus Pauling, who was awarded the 1954 Nobel Prize for chemistry and the 1962 Nobel Prize for peace and who has been the recipient of over 40 honorary degrees from colleges and universities in the United States and abroad wrote in 1985: *"When I discovered, twenty years ago, that the new developments in the field of nutrition were being ignored, I became so interested that most of my effort since that time has been devoted to research and education in this field."* [79]

Dr. Pauling noted 1985 in his book "How to Live Longer and Feel Better": *"I am, for example, impressed by the fact that the Committee on the Feeding of Laboratory Animals of the U.S. National Academy of Sciences / National Research Council recommends far more vitamin C for monkeys than the Food and Nutrition Board of the same U.S. National Academy of Sciences / National Research Council recommends for human beings."* [79] The amount of vitamin C recommended for monkeys, whose body chemistry is very similar to that of humans, is 55 milligrams per kilogram body weight. [146] This is 3850 milligrams for a human adult of 155 pounds (70 kilograms) body weight.

Vitamin C is an essential biochemical tool for the production and protection of collagen that forms the connective tissue including blood vessel walls. When the vitamin C level is high, the body can manufacture high-quality collagen in sufficient quantities. [74] All mechanisms known today leading to cardiovascular disease can be triggered by vitamin C deficiency, as described in detail earlier in this book. [76, 147]

Studies of soldiers killed in the Korean and Vietnam wars showed that nearly 75 percent of the victims at the age of 25 or younger had already developed some form of arteriosclerotic

	All Patients (n=65)		Patients with Starting Coronary Sclerosis* (n=21)	
Age 40-49	5	(9%)	4	(8%)
50-59	24	(44%)	8	(40%)
60-69	26	(47%)	9	(52%)
Smoker	4	(7%)	1	(5%)
Ex-Smoker	36	(65%)	12	(57%)
Diabetic	4	(7%)	0	(0%)
Pancreas Failure	3	(5%)	1	(5%)
Heart Attack	5	(9%)	0	(0%)
Angioplasty Balloon Catheter	2	(4%)	1	(5%)
Use of Medication	27	(49%)	7	(33%)
Use of Vitamin	36	(65%)	15	(71%)

Clinical data of study participants from patient protocol at study onset.

—Rath M, Niedzwiecki A: Nutritional supplement program halts progression of early coronary arteriosclerosis documented by ultrafast computed tomography [148]

*Coronary sclerosis: Arteriosclerosis of the arteries, which supply the heart muscle with fresh blood, leading to a decreasing supply with oxygen and vital nutrients.

Aggressive progression of coronary heart disease without an appropriate vitamin program

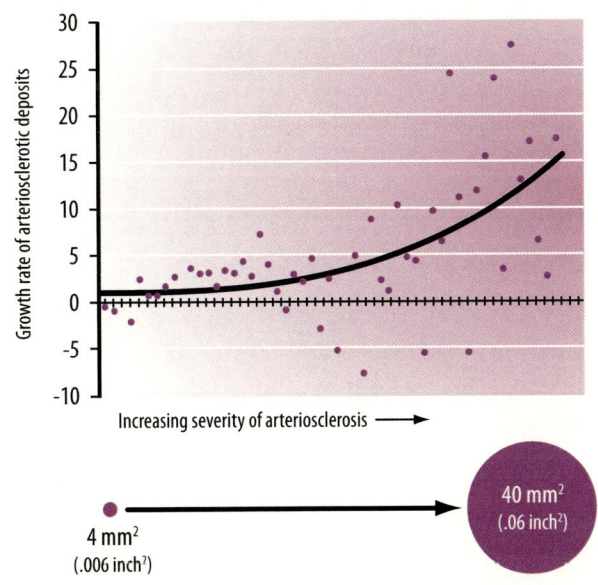

Patients with early coronary heart disease had an average increase in arteriosclerotic plaque (deposit) size of 4 mm² every year (left). The deposits of patients with advanced coronary heart disease increased by 40 mm² or more every year (right). Without an appropriate vitamin program, the arteriosclerotic plaques (deposits) increased very fast with an average growth of 44% every year. This means that without vitamin protection, arteriosclerotic deposits increased approximately half their size every year.

—Rath M, Niedzwiecki A: Nutritional supplement program halts progression of early coronary arteriosclerosis documented by ultrafast computed tomography. [148]

deposits in their arteries. [18] Arteriosclerosis and heart disease are not diseases exclusive to older people.

Without vitamin therapy, coronary heart disease is a very aggressive disease. Deposits in the coronary arteries (the blood tubes that supply the heart muscle with fresh blood) grow, on the average, at a rate of 44 percent per year. This means that without vitamin protection, these deposits that restrict the blood flow increase by approximately half their size every year (see diagram on preceding page). [18, 148]

The result is that every second man and every second woman in our very civilized world still dies from heart attack or stroke to say nothing of the preceding long-time suffering. If we all manage to make this information broadly known, cardiovascular diseases will be almost unknown in future generations.

Dr. Linus Pauling's advice to students: *"When an old and distinguished person speaks to you, listen to him carefully and with respect—but do not believe him. Never put your trust into anything but your own intellect. Your elder, no matter whether he has gray hair or has lost his hair, no matter whether he is a Nobel laureate—may be wrong. The world progresses, year by year, century by century, as the members of the younger generation find out what was wrong among the things that their elders said. So you must always be skeptical—**always think for yourself.**"* (Excerpt from "Linus Pauling: Scientist and Peacemaker", Oregon State University Press 2001). [149]

NATURAL PREVENTION OF ARTERIOSCLEROSIS AND CARDIOVASCULAR DISEASE

The foundation for the prevention of arteriosclerosis is a *continuous and sufficient supply to the cells of the arterial walls with the biochemical tools that they need for a multitude of biochemical tasks.* These 'tools' include vitamins, minerals, trace elements, and other vital cellular nutrients.

First among these is a continuous and sufficient supply of vitamin C which, as mentioned earlier, the human body is unable to manufacture itself, due to a genetic defect. Vitamin C is the indispensable biochemical tool we need to produce strong and elastic connective tissue—the main building block of the arterial walls. Because of this vital function, almost all other mammals manufacture vitamin C in considerable quantities.

The human body depends utterly for its maintenance on a sufficient and continuous dietary intake of vitamin C and other cellular nutrients. The following table lists the various important nutrients for cells. [10, 18, 24, 148] The lower amounts represent the minimum daily amounts that a healthy adult should take for optimum cardiovascular health and to prevent cardiovascular disease. The higher numbers show to what level the daily dosage could be increased if there is an increased need. Every adult should take at least the lower amounts to prevent heart attack or stroke. Those with a family history of heart attack should take more. And those who have suffered a heart attack or stroke should take even more.

VITAMINS

Beta-carotene + natural carotenoids .... 5 -   20 mg
Vitamin A .... 2000 - 10000 I.U.
Vitamin B1 (Thiamine) .... 10 -   300 mg
Vitamin B2 (Riboflavin) .... 10 -   100 mg
Vitamin B3 (Nicotinate) .... 50 -   500 mg
Vitamin B5 (Pantothenate) .... 50 -   200 mg
Vitamin B6 (Pyridoxine) .... 15 -   250 mg
Vitamin B12 (Cyanocobalamin) .... 25 - 2500 mcg
Biotin .... 100 -   500 mcg
Folic Acid .... 350 - 5000 mcg
Inositol .... 30 -   150 mg
Vitamin C .... 2000 - 15000 mg or more
Vitamin D3 .... 1000 - 3000 I.U.
Vitamin E (d-alpha-, d-beta-, d-gamma-, d-delta-Tocopherols and -Tocotrienols) .... 150 -   1000 I.U.

MINERALS

Calcium	200 - 800 mg
Magnesium	100 - 400 mg
Phosphate	10 - 60 mg
Potassium	50 - 500 mg

TRACE ELEMENTS

Chromium	50 - 200 mcg
Copper	300 - 2000 mcg
Manganese	2 - 10 mg
Molybdenum	60 - 300 mcg
Selenium	100 - 300 mcg
Zinc	5 - 30 mg

OTHER IMPORTANT CELL NUTRIENTS

Bioflavonoids	100 - 1000 mg
Coenzyme Q10	30 - 300 mg
Alpha Lipoic Acid	200 - 1200 mg
L-Arginine	40 - 4000 mg
L-Carnitine	30 - 3000 mg
L-Cysteine	50 - 500 mg
L-Lysine	100 - 6000 mg
L-Proline	100 - 3000 mg
Taurine	30 - 4000 mg
Omega 3 Fatty Acids	500 - 6000 mg
Pine Bark - Grape Seed Extract	10 - 50 mg

It would seem that a person would need to take as many as 33 different vitamin supplement tablets several times a day for optimum cardiovascular health and to prevent cardiovascular disease. This is not the case. With a good vitamin formula, many of these nutrients can be effectively combined for optimum result.

Optimum cardiovascular health depends on an optimum functioning of endothelial cells (cells coating the inside of the blood vessels), myocardial cells (heart muscle cells), smooth muscle cells (muscle cells regulating the diameter of the blood vessels), macrophages (defense cells), and other cell systems.

Optimum metabolic function of these cells depends on the availability of the essential biochemical tools listed above. This not only helps protect the blood vessels but also improves heart function. [76, 150]

EFFECTIVE NATURAL TREATMENT OF ARTERIOSCLEROSIS AND CARDIOVASCULAR DISEASE

To break down already existing arteriosclerosis, a true healing process must begin in the arterial wall.

The arterial wall has become diseased due to chronic vitamin deficiency. The most important vitamin for the arterial wall is vitamin C. It enables and stimulates the muscle cells in the arterial wall to manufacture properly functioning collagen molecules, thus restoring and maintaining a strong and elastic arterial wall. But other micronutrients are also of vital importance as biochemical tools for this healing process, especially to decompose and remove the deposits of repair particles—the arteriosclerotic plaques—from the arterial walls. [151, 152]

The Natural Healing of Arteriosclerosis

1

Lysine and Proline plus Vitamin C rebuild stable collagen and thus re-stabilize the arterial wall. Hence, substitutional repair processes that built up arteriosclerotic plaques become unnecessary and repair particles like Lp(a) are no longer needed in the arterial wall.

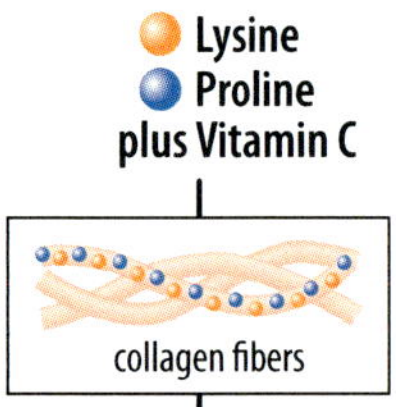

● Lysine
● Proline
plus Vitamin C

collagen fibers

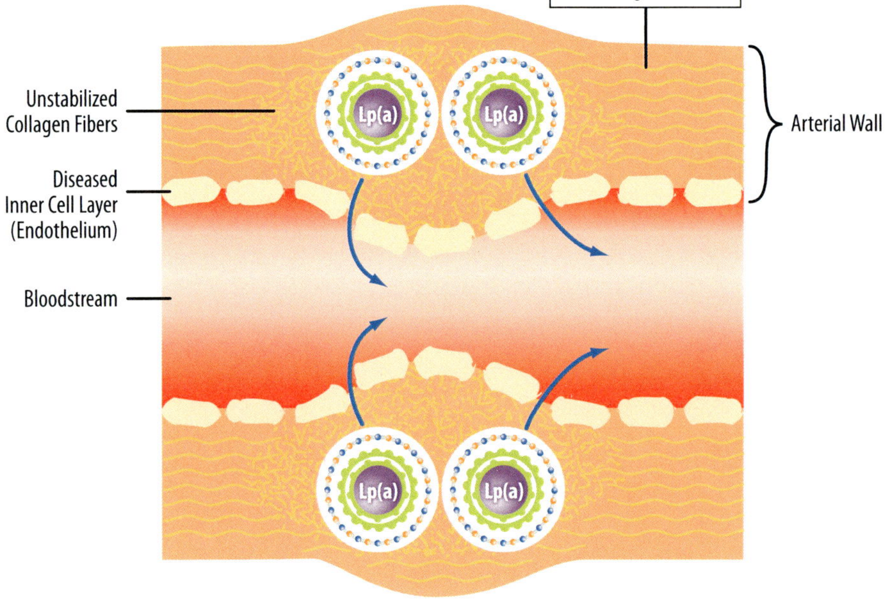

Unstabilized Collagen Fibers

Arterial Wall

Diseased Inner Cell Layer (Endothelium)

Bloodstream

Lp(a) Lp(a)

Lp(a) Lp(a)

Lysine and Proline put a Teflon-like layer around the adhesive Lp(a) particles, neutralize their adhesiveness and are thus able to prevent further growth of arteriosclerotic plaques and to reduce existing plaques.

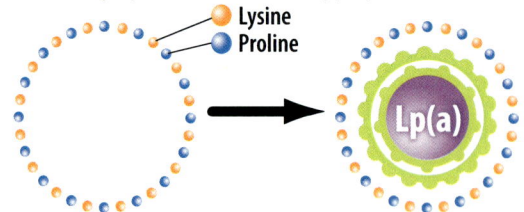

● Lysine
● Proline

Lp(a)

2 Vitamin C and Vitamin E reduce the overgrowth of arterial muscle cells and allow the endothelium cells to recover.

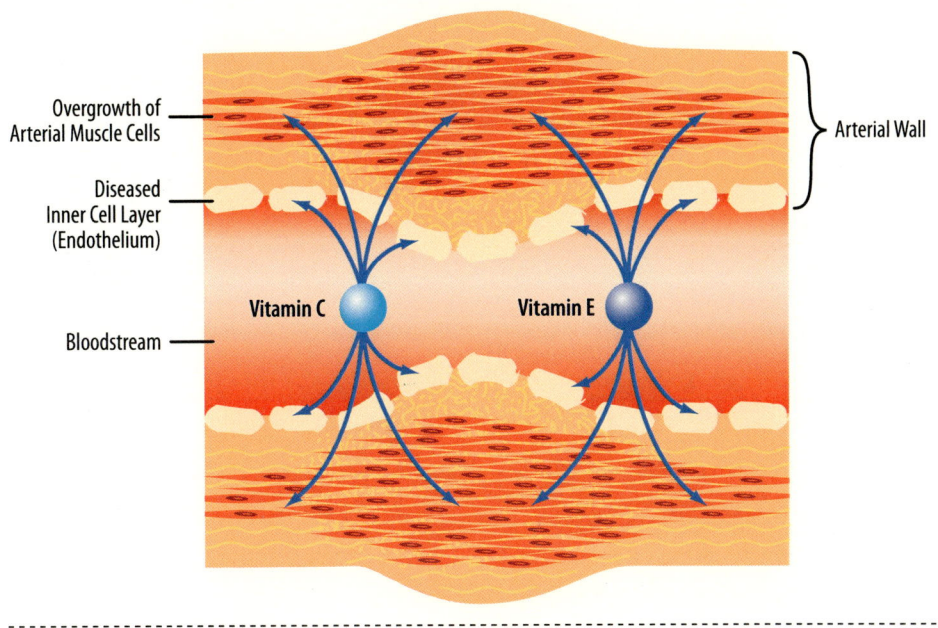

Overgrowth of Arterial Muscle Cells

Diseased Inner Cell Layer (Endothelium)

Bloodstream

Vitamin C

Vitamin E

Arterial Wall

3 The collagen fibers, arterial muscle cells and endothelium cells are restored, and the arterial wall functions normally.

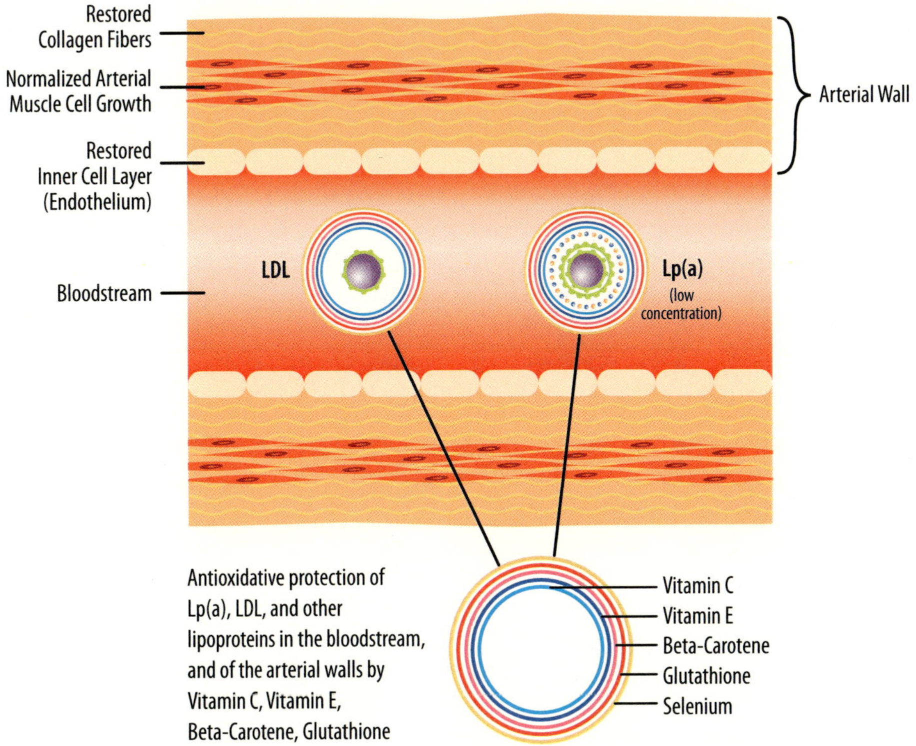

Restored Collagen Fibers

Normalized Arterial Muscle Cell Growth

Restored Inner Cell Layer (Endothelium)

Bloodstream

Arterial Wall

LDL

Lp(a) (low concentration)

Antioxidative protection of Lp(a), LDL, and other lipoproteins in the bloodstream, and of the arterial walls by Vitamin C, Vitamin E, Beta-Carotene, Glutathione and Selenium.

Vitamin C
Vitamin E
Beta-Carotene
Glutathione
Selenium

For patients with existing cardiovascular disease or who have a high risk for cardiovascular disease, the cellular nutrients listed above are recommended. But in particular the following nutrients should be taken in higher dosages [18, 148]:

- **Vitamin C** for the protection and natural healing of the arterial wall, and decomposition of arteriosclerotic plaques.

- **Vitamin D** for optimization of calcium metabolism and decomposition of calcium deposits in the arterial wall.

- **Vitamin E** for antioxidative protection of cells and tissues.

- **Folic acid**, **vitamin B6** and **vitamin B12** for protective function against homocysteine.

- **Copper** for stability of the arterial wall by networking collagen molecules.

- **L-Lysine** for collagen production, stability of arterial wall and decomposition of plaques.

- **L-Proline** for collagen production, stability of arterial wall and decomposition of plaques.

- **L-Arginine** for dilatation of arteries and normalization of blood platelet aggregation. [153 - 157]

- **Pinebark extract** supports vitamin C function and contributes to the stability of arterial walls.

In addition, the following nutrients should be used:

- **Betaine** for protective function against homocysteine by breaking it down further (together with vitamin B6, vitamin B12, and folic acid).

- **Chondroitin sulfate** and **N-acetyl-glucosamine** as connective tissue components ('cement') for the stability of the arterial wall.

The amino acids lysine and proline compete against constituents of the blood-vessel walls and against constituents of arteriosclerotic lesions for the binding of Lp(a). If the binding sites of Lp(a) are saturated with lysine and proline, Lp(a) can no longer bind to the blood-vessel walls. Similar to a Teflon layer around the Lp(a) particle, lysine and proline prevent the Lp(a) particle from attaching to the blood-vessel wall. In this way, the therapeutic use of these two amino acids prevents further buildup of Lp(a) in these walls. More importantly, optimum concentrations of lysine and proline release from the blood-vessel wall already deposited Lp(a) and other lipoproteins. [76]

Combining these substances with vitamin C is ideal. Vitamin C reduces the need for further Lp(a) deposits in the vascular wall, and the Lp(a) binding inhibitors lysine and proline increase the release of already deposited Lp(a). [75, 158, 159, 160]

The blood stream transports the detached Lp(a) molecules to the liver where they are broken down. By gradually discharging the lipoproteins from the arteriosclerotic deposits, the deposits are dismantled and blood circulation improves. This is a natural process where molecule after molecule is discharged from the arterial wall and then immediately broken down by the liver. Complications like detachment of plaques as seen during balloon catheter angioplasty (an artificial widening of an artery from its inside by means of a tube with an expandable balloon) do not occur.

ON THE REVERSAL AND PREVENTION
OF HEART DISEASE, TWO CASE HISTORIES

The following two case histories show the immediate success of Dr. Linus Pauling's and Dr. Matthias Rath's drug-free therapy of terminally ill patients with advanced heart disease. [158] This therapy consists of the common nutritional supplements described earlier, in specified ratios, taken at home (see pages 47-48). Of course, a physician should monitor the progress and perform standard tests to determine if other risk factors, deficiencies, etc. exist and to make sure that they are not overlooked. Here is a summary of Dr. Pauling's first case, followed by a second patient who had the same rapid and remarkable recovery that appears to be the usual response to his regimen:

In March 1991, a 71 year old CAD (coronary artery disease, the coronary arteries are the arteries which supply the heart muscle with blood) patient, whose condition had inexorably worsened for 33 years despite three heart bypasses and other surgery, was informed that most of his blood vessels were clogged, but that he could not have additional surgery. In May, with steadily increasing pain and deterioration of his health, he elected to begin Dr. Pauling's and Dr. Rath's lysine / vitamin C dietary therapy, starting with a low dose. By mid June, he was taking the normal 5 to 6 grams of lysine and other essential nutrients. By July, he was free of angina pectoris (pain) and could even walk two miles and do yard work without discomfort. In August, he cut up a tree with a chain saw, and then started painting his house. By October 1991, he was free of all symptoms of disease and was able to reduce the nutrient dosing to a maintenance level, which all such patients should continue for life.

In May 2002, a 56-year-old heart disease patient reported that, after using Dr. Pauling's method, he had just recovered from a terminal, hopeless condition. He had endured 10 years of continuous angina pectoris (a symptom of coronary artery disease caused by diminished supply of blood to the heart muscle marked by sharp chest pains and a feeling of being suffocated) and many heart attacks while his CAD steadily worsened after conventional therapy that included four bypasses. In June 2001, he had experienced extreme pain during another heart attack and was told his disease had progressed to a point where it was now inoperable. Two of the four bypasses were completely blocked and a third graft was partially blocked. He found vitamin therapy, took daily 14 grams of vitamin C, 6 grams of lysine as well as the other supplements mentioned earlier. In only two days he felt markedly better and began jogging, free of pain and other symptoms. [161]

DIET AND EXERCISE

A diet rich in vegetables and fruits and low in sugars and animal fats promotes cardiovascular health. Regular physical activity is another precondition for cardiovascular health: Moderate, regular exercise such as walking or bicycling is ideal. It is something that anyone can perform. [18]

CESSATION OF SMOKING

A large number of scientific studies with smokers reveal that the more cigarettes that are smoked, the lower the blood concentration of vitamin C. Ten cigarettes per day decreased vitamin C blood levels by about 30%; 20 cigarettes per day decreased vitamin C blood levels by approximately 40%. [162] Vitamin C is used up capturing and neutralizing the toxic substances found in tobacco smoke. One single cigarette uses up approximately 25 milligrams of vitamin C. This decrease of vitamin C worsens the blood vessel wall maintenance and thus increases the risk for cardiovascular and peripheral vascular disease. [75]

—13—

Remedies for High Blood Pressure (Hypertension)

Hundreds of millions of people worldwide suffer from high blood pressure (known in medical terms as hypertension or hypertonia). It is the single largest epidemic of all cardiovascular diseases. [18] Systolic pressures (blood pressure peaks caused by the normal contraction of the heart) of 140 mm Hg ("mm Hg" is a measuring unit of pressure) and diastolic pressures (the blood pressure in the arteries when the heart is relaxed) of 90 mm Hg are generally regarded as the upper limits of normal blood pressure.

In diagnosis, if the cause of a person's hypertension can be established, the hypertensive state is called *"secondary" hypertension*. This means that it occurs secondary to some other known disorder. If no specific cause for the hypertension can be discerned, the hypertension is designated as *"essential"* or *"primary" hypertension*. The terms "essential" or "primary", translated to less esoteric language, mean "we do not know the cause". [163]

The so-called "essential" hypertension comprises approximately 80% of all cases of high blood pressure. [164]

Cellular lack of essential nutrients leads to thickened and less elastic arterial walls (arteriosclerosis) and to an increased vascular wall tension. Due to this the blood pressure is increased.

An increased blood pressure, through the increased strain put on the arterial wall, accelerates the formation and progression of arteriosclerosis.

The tension of the vascular wall in particular is increased by a lack of natural relaxing factors normally produced in sufficient amounts by the cells covering the inside of the artery (endothelium cells), and it is decreased by a sufficient availability of relaxing factors.

Optimum daily nutrients to handle a high blood pressure condition especially include:

- Vitamin C
- Lipoic acid
- L-Arginine
- Magnesium
- Calcium
- Vitamin E
- Coenzyme Q10
- L-Lysine
- L-Proline

These substances are included on the list of nutrients on pages 47-48, but are especially vital in providing cells with the biochemical tools they need in order to remedy a high blood pressure condition, together with the other nutrients on that list. This program should be supervised by a doctor, who needs to monitor the blood pressure regularly and to adjust accordingly any medication the patient is taking. Otherwise, the blood pressure can easily drop too low.

Vitamin C and **lipoic acid**:   A number of clinical studies have found that vitamin C promotes vasodilation (relaxation of the arteries), probably through its effect on the generation of nitric oxide, a signaling molecule that induces the relaxation of vascular smooth muscle cells and also inhibits platelet aggregation. Nitric oxide is a potent vasodilatative factor.   Another name for nitric oxide is EDRF (endothelium-derived relaxing factor). In this study, published by an international research team at the Oregon State University in 2002, the authors reported that lipoic acid and vitamin C enhanced nitric oxide production in cultured vascular endothelial cells. Vitamin C enhances nitric oxide synthesis by stabilizing and increasing the amount of a molecule named tetrahydrobiopterin critical to the synthesis of nitric oxide, but the mechanism by which lipoic acid stimulates the production of nitric oxide remains unknown. [147, 165, 166]

Vitamin C also increases the production of prostacyclin, a vasodilating (blood vessel widening) hormone. [75]

L-Arginine: The endothelium cells produce one molecule of EDRF (endothelium-derived relaxing factor or nitric oxide) from one molecule of L-arginine. [75, 167]

Magnesium: This mineral is essential for the activation of approximately 300 enzymes (biochemical tools) in the human body. Magnesium is a potent natural vasodilator (artery wall relaxant). If there is a lack of magnesium, more calcium streams into the blood-vessel muscle cells, making them more prone to contract and also increasing the blood-vessel constricting effect of the body's own blood-pressure raising substances. Fifty percent of patients who have low blood levels of magnesium or a general magnesium deficiency, have a high blood pressure. Their blood pressure is usually easily normalized by magnesium supplementation. [168 - 176]

A magnesium deficiency is very common, for the following reasons:

- Artificial fertilizers used to grow grains, fruits and vegetables very often do not contain any magnesium thus leading to a magnesium-deficient diet. [173, 177]

- Caffeine (found in coffee, cola beverages, etc.) increases magnesium excretion via the kidneys. [177, 178]

- Too much sugar—such as found in most soft drinks—increases metabolic magnesium consumption and magnesium excretion via the kidneys. [179, 180]

- High dietary protein intake increases metabolic magnesium consumption. [181]

Calcium optimizes mineral metabolism, decreases artery wall tension and lowers elevated blood pressure. [18, 182, 183, 184]

Vitamin E is an important antioxidant that protects all cell membranes (the walls of cells). For cardiovascular disease, this is especially important for the cells on the inside of the blood vessels (the endothelium cells). Vitamin E also protects blood components such as lipoproteins. [185, 186]

Coenzyme Q10 plays a key role in the mitochondria, the power stations inside the cells that produce energy. [187] Moreover, it protects the membranes (walls) of the cells and the membranes of their organelles; an organelle is a minute specialized part of a cell. [188] Coenzyme Q10 helps, in a natural way, to lower high blood pressure by 10 to 15 percent in the majority of cases. [189 - 200]

L-lysine and **L-proline** release deposited Lp(a) (lipoprotein(a)) as well as other lipoproteins from the vascular wall. [76] The combination of these substances with **vitamin C** may be considered ideal since vitamin C reduces the need for further Lp(a) deposition in the vascular wall and the natural inhibitors L-lysine and L-proline enhance the release of already deposited Lp(a). [75, 158, 159, 160]

Another natural substance that also has been found to lower high blood pressure is **garlic**. [201]

Another cause of high blood pressure is an excess storage of protein. If you continuously eat more calories and more protein than you need, the surplus protein is stored on the outside of the walls of the body's capillaries, the smallest of our blood vessels that have diameters the size of a single hair. This leads to a thickening of the capillary wall that makes it less permeable (less penetrable). Fewer nutrients then pass from the blood through to cells where they are needed. In an effort to maintain a sufficient supply of nutrients through the thickened capillary walls, the pressure in the capillaries increases, leading to hypertension (high blood pressure).

Overweight and an excess of proteins in the blood are the diagnostic criteria of this condition. To handle, it is important to reduce the dietary protein intake. Going on a vegetarian diet for some weeks is the slower way to do this. A fasting program (supervised by a doctor) achieves the result more quickly. In this way the increased thickness of the capillary walls and the resulting high blood pressure can be normalized if it was caused by a continuous intake of too many calories with a high proportion of proteins. [202, 202A]

—14—

Heart Failure

We are in the midst of a congestive heart failure epidemic in the United States. Approximately 4.8 millions of Americans are diagnosed with congestive heart failure (CHF). Each year, there are an estimated 400,000 new cases of CHF. Half of those patients will die within 5 years. [25]

Cardiomyopathy—which means "heart muscle disease"—or heart failure, or congestive heart failure (CHF), is a deficiency disease of the heart muscle characterized by decreasing contractive performance, enlargement of the heart chambers, and impaired blood circulation in different organs of the body, including the kidneys. The term "congestive" means "with congestion"— a congestion (accumulation) of blood in the enlarged heart.

The symptoms of this illness are shortness of breath, exhaustion, and edema (an abnormal accumulation of watery fluid in the tissues or cavities of the body, often causing visible swelling). More than 15 million people worldwide suffer from this.

The current term for this disease is, in the majority of cases, "idiopathic cardiomyopathy". This sounds impressive, but translated to a less esoteric language, the word "idiopathic" means "we do not know the cause".

The heart is one of the most metabolically active organs in the body, pumping approximately 2000 gallons of blood through 65,000 miles of blood vessels, beating 100,000 times each day (American Heart Association 2002). In order to cope with this heavy workload the heart needs sufficient supplies of "cell fuel".

A healthy heart has the highest magnesium, carnitine and coenzyme Q10 contents of any organ. [10] Only the liver—the central biochemical laboratory of the body—has a similarly high content of coenzyme Q10. Ninety-five percent of all body energy producing metabolic processes depend on the presence of coenzyme Q10.

Coenzyme Q10 concentrations in tissues decrease with age: The heart of a 40 year old contains only 68 percent and the heart of someone who is 79 years old contains only 42 percent of the Q10 of a 20 years old person.

Our modern food supply usually does not contain sufficient amounts of essential cellular nutrients. Thus deficiencies develop. First and foremost, this is fatal for the hard-working heart muscle—100,000 contractions every 24 hours.

Moreover, cholesterol-lowering drugs — being absolutely unnecessary since vitamin C does the same job much better and without side effects [203, 204]—increase Lp(a) [205], thus promoting arteriosclerosis and markedly increasing the probability of heart attack or stroke [206, 207]. Such drugs also decrease coenzyme Q10 [208], thus promoting heart failure. Dr. Peter Langsjoen, a cardiologist and researcher at the University of Texas Health Center, reports "a frightening increase in heart failure secondary to statin usage" [25, 27]. Cholesterol-lowering statin drugs include widely used brands such as Lipitor® (atorvastatin), Zocor® (simvastatin), Pravachol® (pravastatin), Lescol® (fluvastatin), Mevacor® (lovastatin), Crestor® (rosuvastatin).

The common treatment of an existing heart failure that use diuretics (drugs that remove excessive water from tissues) worsens the disease. Even more vital nutrients—water-soluble vitamins, minerals, trace elements—are flushed out of the body, worsening the nutrient deficiency that had been the original cause of the condition. Every second patient who has been diagnosed with congestive heart failure dies within five years.

A better choice is to use a natural health program described earlier that corrects cardiovascular disease. Such program should be supervised by a responsible physician. Vitamins B1 [209], B2, B5, B6, B12, biotin, niacin (vitamin B3), vitamin C, vitamin E, coenzyme Q10 [210 - 216], carnitine [217 - 219] and taurine [220] increase the pumping ability of the heart, normalize enlarged heart chambers, decrease edema and shortness of breath. As a result, physical performance and life expectancy increase markedly.

The amino acid arginine helps improve circulation in CHF (congestive heart failure) patients. [221]

Magnesium deficiency is frequently associated with CHF, and can cause heart arrhythmia, an irregular heartbeat. Taking supplemental magnesium can decrease the occurrence of arrhythmia. [222] Magnesium is especially effective when taken in combination with potassium. [223]

Extract from Hawthorn berries is extremely effective in the treatment of early-stage heart failure. [224] It increases blood flow and heart strength, and acts as a protective antioxidant. [225, 226]

—15—

Nutrition After a Heart Attack

There are several natural cellular nutrients that have powerful effects preventing blood clotting and dissolving blood clots—without dangerous side effects:

Vitamin C has anti-coagulative (preventing blood clotting) and profibrinolytic (dissolving fibrin, the glue that holds blood clots together) properties. It normalizes blood platelet adhesiveness and blood platelet aggregation (clotting). [75, 227]

Functions of **vitamin E** that are important in protecting against coronary heart disease and peripheral vascular disease include protecting LDL (low-density lipoprotein) cholesterol against deterioration, maintaining or improving the function of the cells on the interior surface of blood vessels, inhibiting an increase in quantity of smooth muscle cells and inhibiting adhesion and aggregation (clotting) of blood platelets. [228] As a note, the form of vitamin E that is called d-alpha-tocopherol is the most beneficial form of vitamin E for the cells. [229 - 233]

Endothelium-derived relaxing factor (EDRF) has an inhibiting effect on blood platelet aggregation (clotting). **N-acetylcysteine** intensifies this inhibiting effect. [234]

Coenzyme Q10 can provide rapid protective effects in patients with acute myocardial infarction if administered within 3 days of the onset of symptoms. [235]

For the basic treatment of cardiovascular disease, please see chapter 12, How to Prevent and Reverse Heart Disease.

Don't Take Aspirin:
The Side Effects of Pharmaceutical Drugs

The painkiller aspirin is routinely prescribed to everyone who has had a heart attack or stroke. Moreover, aspirin is now taken by 50 million healthy US citizens under the illusion it will prevent heart attacks.

> *"The remedy is worse than the disease."*
> — SIR FRANCIS BACON
> British philosopher, essayist, statesman, 1561-1626

Aspirin is supposed to inhibit blood clotting, more exactly the aggregation of blood platelets, in order that in the narrowed coronary arteries no further clots develop. Such clots would otherwise interrupt blood circulation and cause another myocardial infarction (interruption of blood supply and heart attack), this time of another area of the heart muscle.

Unfortunately, aspirin also hinders the production of collagen and elastin fibers—the exact fibers that provide and maintain stability and elasticity of the arterial walls, including the walls of the coronary (heart) arteries.

Primarily because of a chronic vitamin C deficiency, the body is unable to produce sufficient stable collagen. It is exactly this lack of vital building material that leads to the cracks in the arterial walls that the body, on an emergency basis, repairs with molecules produced by the liver: mainly fibrin and lipoprotein(a).

Such continuous emergency repair, that we call arteriosclerosis, eventually leads to increased deposits and a reduced inner arterial diameter. A small blood clot is then sufficient in order to completely interrupt the supply of blood, thereby of oxygen and vital cellular nutrients, especially in the relatively small coronary (heart) arteries.

The part of the heart muscle that was supplied by this coronary artery then dies.

Aspirin is a direct antagonist (counteracting substance) of vitamin C. As described earlier, vitamin C is responsible for the production of sufficient high-grade collagen and thus for healthy arterial walls. But aspirin impedes sufficient collagen production and thus impedes the maintenance and restoration of healthy arterial walls. In this way, long-term use of aspirin *prevents* the recovery of the vascular (blood vessel) system. Arterial lesions do not heal, but progress. The risk of further interruptions to the blood supply (infarctions) increases, in the heart or in the brain, thus leading to heart attack or stroke, as well as the risk of other diseases such as stomach ulcers and gastrointestinal bleeding. [236, 237]

According to a study published in the January, 2004, issue of the Journal of the National Cancer Institute, regular use of aspirin for 20 years or more may be associated with an increased risk of pancreatic cancer in women, *the fourth leading cause of cancer-related deaths in the United States*. Researchers at Harvard University found that women who reported more than 20 years of regular aspirin use had a 58% increased risk of pancreatic cancer compared with women who never regularly consumed more than two aspirin tablets per week. When the investigators compared women who had reported consistent, regular aspirin use with women who were non-users during the same time period, they found that the risk of pancreatic cancer increased with the increasing aspirin dose. Compared with non-users, women who took 14 or more aspirin tablets per week had an 86 percent increased risk of pancreatic cancer. [238]

Vitamin C, Vitamin E, Arginine and Cysteine or Acetylcysteine normalize an increased tendency of the blood platelets to form blood clots—naturally and without side effects. [156, 227, 234, 239, 240, 241]

Dr. Matthias Rath explains, "*The long-term side effects of the most common medicaments are willfully concealed or trivialized. As long-*

term use of these medicaments makes ill the pharmaceutical industry in this way purposefully creates markets for new pharmaceuticals, with sales in the range of billions of dollars." [242]

What kills more Americans every year than World War II and the Vietnam War combined?

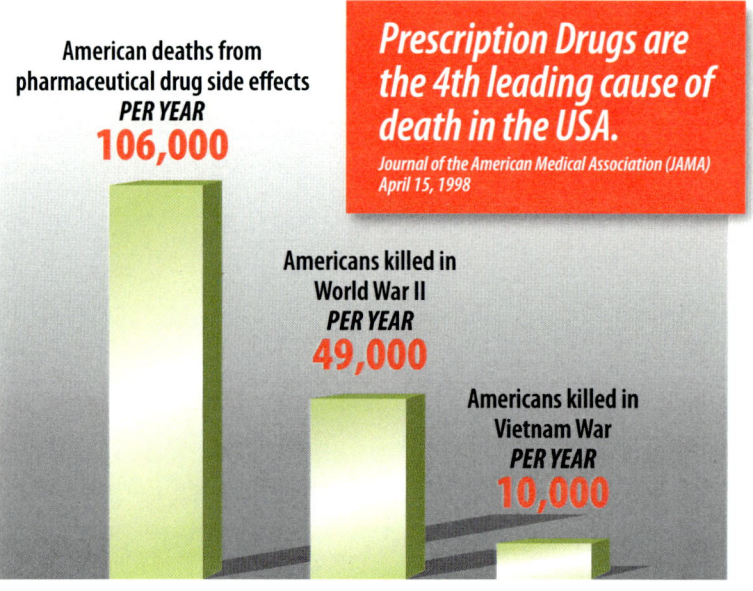

American deaths from pharmaceutical drug side effects
PER YEAR
106,000

Prescription Drugs are the 4th leading cause of death in the USA.
Journal of the American Medical Association (JAMA)
April 15, 1998

Americans killed in
World War II
PER YEAR
49,000

Americans killed in
Vietnam War
PER YEAR
10,000

[243]

In 2001, the top 10 pharmaceutical companies each had sales of more than $11 billion. Together, they generated $172 billion in sales, more than 59 percent of the total for all 50 pharmaceutical companies. They also marketed a combined total of 23 products, each of which brought in more than $1 billion in sales. [244]

On June 23rd, 1997, Fortune magazine, one of the major Wall Street weeklies, carried an article about the health care system. It contained an interview with an investment consultant for pharmaceutical companies who claimed that "everyone loses if [disease] eradication therapy catches on". [245, 246]

The world-famous American psychiatrist Carl C. Pfeiffer who successfully treated more than 10,000 cases of insanity by administering appropriate amounts of natural cellular nutrients stated, *"Generally, the use of drugs is a self-deception which sacrifices long-term health for immediate results."* [247]

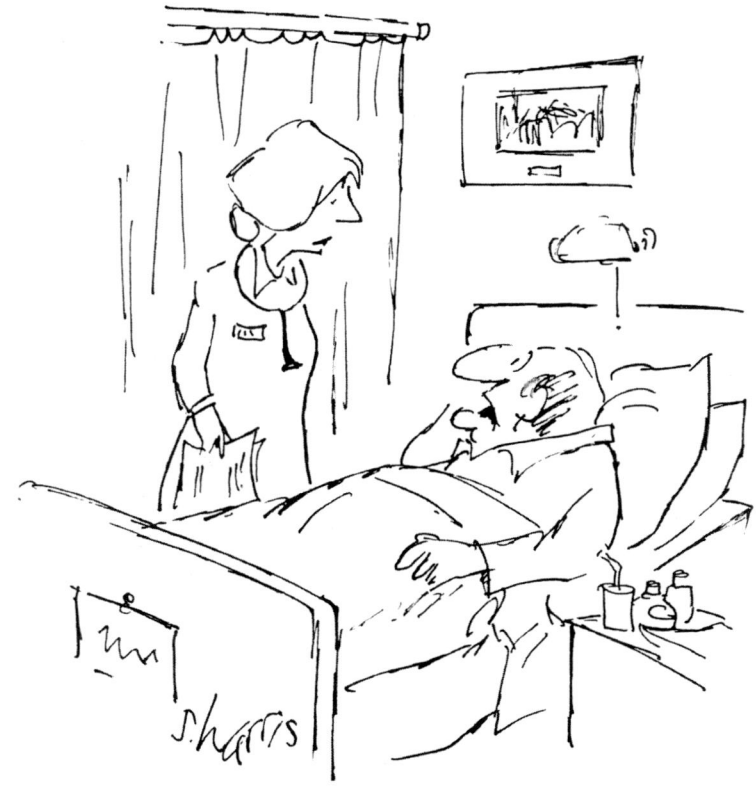

"I stopped taking the medicine because I prefer
the original disease to the side effects."

SUMMARY

Apart from water, 50% of the body is formed by structural tissue named collagen that maintains the body's form, stabilizes the bones and holds the organs in place. The walls of the arteries are made of this structural tissue as well. All structural tissue, including that of the arterial walls, needs to be maintained and for this, a person needs certain biochemical 'tools'. The most important tool for this maintenance is vitamin C. Without it the body cannot make or maintain stable structural tissue including skin, bones, and arteries —and literally the body begins to degenerate and fall apart. And remember, it is not the cholesterol—this is just a marketing scam.

Unfortunately, unlike most animals, the human body cannot manufacture its own vitamin C, and due to modern agricultural processes, chemical fertilizers and pollutants, current food supplies lack sufficient vitamin C content.

Similarly important for the stability and elasticity of all structural tissue in the body, an amino acid called lysine is an essential building substance. Like vitamin C, the body cannot manufacture it, and often current food supplies are deficient as well.

Therefore, in order to maintain a strong and healthy structure throughout the body, including strong arteries, it is vital to take sufficient daily amounts of vitamin C, some lysine and some other natural substances.

But you do not need to take 33 single substances as you might have deduced from the food supplements listed on pages 47-48. A well-composed multi-vitamin product that contains lysine and preferably a non-acidic vitamin C product will keep your arteries and your heart in good health.

If a cardiovascular problem already exists one to two additional food supplement combinations can help to remedy that problem.

—— GLOSSARY ——

Amino acid: A biochemical building block that is connected in chains to form proteins. It consists of carbon, hydrogen, nitrogen, and oxygen. Some amino acids contain also sulfur.

Angina pectoris: A condition of the heart marked by sharp chest pains and a feeling of being suffocated. It is usually a symptom of coronary heart disease brought about by a diminished supply of blood to the heart muscle.

Angiographic: Of or having to do with angiography.

Angiography: Injection of a contrast agent into the blood vessels and following X-ray examination of the blood vessels.

Anti-coagulative: Preventing blood clotting.

Antioxidant: Any substance that prevents oxidation by scavenging oxygen or other aggressive agents.

Anti-oxidative: Preventing oxidation and thus damage through oxidation.

Arrhythmia: An irregular heartbeat.

Arterial: Of or having to do with an artery or arteries.

Arteriosclerosis: A progressive thickening and hardening of the walls of the arteries causing a decrease or loss of circulation.

Arteriosclerotic deposits: Arteriosclerotic plaques.

Arteriosclerotic plaques: Swellings within the artery walls which narrow the artery and thus restrict the blood flow. The swellings are composed of deposited fibrin, lipoprotein(a), calcium, and arterial muscle cells.

Artery: Arteries are the tubes through which all parts of the body are supplied with fresh blood containing oxygen and vital nutrients.

Ascorbic acid: Vitamin C.

Balloon catheter angioplasty: An artificial widening of an artery from its inside by means of a tube with an expandable balloon.

Biochemical: Of or having to do with biochemistry.

Biochemistry: The chemistry of living organisms.

Biosynthesis: The formation of a compound by the chemical union of simpler compounds in a living organism, for example the formation of a protein by the chemical union of amino acids.

Blood vessel: The blood tubes, either supplying blood loaded with oxygen and nutrients to the cells throughout the body (arteries), or returning unloaded blood to the heart and to the lungs (veins).

Bypass surgery: Bridging a narrowed or blocked part of a heart artery by inserting a piece of vein cut out of one leg. These added pieces will themselves frequently become narrowed or blocked after some time as arteriosclerosis develops also in these veins.

Capillary: Any of the smallest blood tubes in the body with a very slender, hairlike opening.

Carbohydrate: Sugar and starch are carbohydrates. Potatoes, wheat, rice, and corn contain much starch.

Cardiac: Of or having to do with the heart: cardiac disease, cardiac arteries.

Cardiomyopathy: This medical term means "heart muscle disease". Please see "congestive heart failure".

Cardiovascular disease (CVD): A progressive thickening and hardening of the walls of the arteries (arteriosclerosis), including the arteries supplying the heart, which decreases circulation in the heart muscle. A loss of circulation in one ore more heart arteries causes a heart attack.

Cell: The extremely small, basic unit of living matter of which all plants and animals are made. A human body contains approximately 50 trillion cells. The human body has blood cells, muscle cells, nerve cells, and other kinds. Cells vary in size and shape but are generally microscopic. Their diameter is 10 to 50 micrometers (millionth of meters). The cells are the biochemical factories of the body assembling and dismantling thousands of different substances.

Cell membranes: The walls of the cells.

Cellular: Of or having to do with cells, concerning the cells, in the cells, etc.

Cholesterol: Cholesterol, a wax-like colorless substance, is one of the most important biochemical building blocks in the body, the biochemical foundation for a huge number of substances without which your body would not be alive. Cholesterol plays a vital part in the structure of every cell (the basic living unit of the body), is a key molecule for building and maintaining the brain cells and all other cells of the nervous system. Too little cholesterol also appears to be related to the onset of Alzheimer's disease. In addition, cholesterol is the mother substance for the body's production of a large number of vitamins and hormones. For example, all female and male sex hormones are made from cholesterol being responsible for fertility, muscular strength, and potency.

Collagen: A fibrous protein that provides stability and strength to blood vessels, bones, cartilages, eyes, heart, skin, teeth, tendons, and, in fact, essentially to all parts of the body.

Congestive: With congestion, with a blood congestion, with retention of blood in the heart.

Congestive heart failure (CHF): Heart failure or congestive heart failure or cardiomyopathy (meaning "heart muscle disease") is a deficiency disease of the heart muscle characterized by decreasing contractive performance, enlargement of heart chambers, and impaired blood circulation in different organs of the body including the kidneys. The symptoms are shortness of breath, edema and exhaustion. More than 15 million people worldwide suffer from this disease.

Connective tissue: At least 30 percent of the tissues in the body do not consist of organs, such as lungs, liver, kidneys, etc., but of a network of strong collagen and elastic (elastin) fibers forming the connective tissue or extracellular matrix. This is the structural tissue that holds your body together, maintains its form, maintains the form of the organs and holds them in place. Connective tissue is also the main building material of the artery walls, which gives the arteries stability and elasticity and thus keeps them healthy. Moreover, throughout the body, the connective tissue transports nutrients from the capillaries to the cells of the organs, transports waste products from the cells to the capillaries and lymphatic vessels, acts as a macromolecular filter protecting the cells against pollutants and has vital defense functions against invaders, such as bacteria or viruses.

Contract: To make smaller; shrink; shorten: to contract a muscle.

Contractility: The ability of the heart muscle to contract and thus pump blood through the blood tubes of the body.

Contractive: Of or having to do with contraction.

Coronary arteries: The blood vessels (tubes) supplying the heart muscle with fresh blood, including oxygen and nutrients.

Coronary artery disease (CAD): Progressive arteriosclerosis in the coronary (heart) arteries causing a decrease of circulation in the heart muscle. A loss of circulation causes heart attack.

Coronary heart disease (CHD): Progressive arteriosclerosis in the coronary (heart) arteries causing a decrease of circulation in the heart muscle. A loss of circulation causes heart attack.

Diastolic blood pressure: The diastolic pressure is the pressure in the arteries when the heart is relaxed.

Diuretic: Any drug extracting water from the body in order to remove edema from legs, lungs, etc. Diuretics leach out also vital nutrients.

Edema: An abnormal accumulation of watery fluid in the tissues or cavities of the body, often causing visible swelling.

Endothelium-derived relaxing factor (EDRF): The endothelium cells produce one molecule of EDRF from one molecule of the amino acid L-arginine. EDRF is nitric oxide. It is used as a messenger substance. It effects are: relaxation of the arterial walls thereby increasing the arterial diameter, increasing blood circulation, and reducing high blood pressure.

Endothelial: Of or having to do with the endothelium.

Endothelium: The inner coat of an artery consisting of cells, named endothelium cells.

Enzyme: An enzyme is a protein that serves as a biochemical tool. Numerous enzymes exist in the biochemical 'tool box' of an organism. There may be as many as fifty thousand different kinds of enzymes in a single human body. The building of strong muscles, maintaining smooth elastic hair, nails and skin, detoxifying alcohol and other aggressive substances, killing bacteria, obtaining energy from food, in short, every biochemical process in the body that enables the body to live is performed by enzymes.

Epidemic: Noun: The rapid spreading of a disease so that many people have it at the same time. Adjective: Affecting many people at the same time, widespread.

Fatty acid: Different fatty acids together with glycerine form nutritional fats such as butter or vegetable oils.

Fibrin: A blood protein involved in forming blood clots. Also involved in forming arteriosclerotic plaques.

Fibrinogen: A preliminary form of fibrin.

Fibrinolytic: Dissolving fibrin and thus blood clots.

Genetic defect: An error or an omission in one of the genes. The genes are the body's biochemical 'design specification' and 'work instruction' sheets located in the cells.

Genetic disease: A disease caused by an error or an omission in one of the genes. The genes are the body's biochemical design specification and work instruction sheets (blue prints) located in the cells.

HDL: High density lipoprotein is a heavier lipoprotein particle. It is a carrier protein that consists of approximately 50 percent protein (carrier), 22 percent phospholipids (binder), 20 percent cholesterol (cargo) and 8 percent triglycerides (cargo). It loads cholesterol taken up from food or given off by the cells, and transports it to the liver.

Heart attack: A sudden failure of the heart to function properly that is caused by a loss of circulation in a part of the heart muscle, frequently leading to death.

Heart disease: Progressive arteriosclerosis causing a decrease of circulation in the heart muscle. A loss of circulation causes heart attack.

High blood pressure (hypertonia, hypertension): Of all cardiovascular disease conditions, this is the single largest epidemic. Systolic pressures (pressure peaks caused by contractions of the heart) of 140 mm Hg and diastolic pressures (the diastolic pressure is that in the arteries when the heart is relaxed) of 90 mm Hg are generally regarded as the upper limits of normal blood pressure; "mm Hg" is a measuring unit of pressure referring to a column of mercury that becomes longer or shorter depending on the pressure.

Homocysteine: A harmful decomposition product of the amino acid methionine. Normally the homocysteine blood levels are low. But if its decomposition is impeded— usually because of a lack of biochemical tools such as vitamins B2, B6, B12, and folic acid— homocysteine accumulates. Elevated homocysteine levels are accompanied by an increased risk of arteriosclerotic deterioration of the blood vessel walls.

Hormone: A biochemical substance controlling cell and tissue functions.

Hydroxylation: To connect a group of oxygen and hydrogen to a compound.

Hypertension: High blood pressure.

Hypertonia: High blood pressure.

Inhibitor: Any substance that slows down or hinders a chemical reaction.

Infarction: See "myocardial infarction".

Inverse correlation: Opposite mutual relation of two or more things.

Ischemia: Shortfall in blood supply, for example in the heart arteries due to arteriosclerosis.

Ischemic: Of or having to do with ischemia.

LDL: Low density lipoprotein is a lighter lipoprotein particle. It is a carrier protein and consists approximately of 21 percent protein (carrier), 25 percent phospholipids (binder), 45 percent cholesterol (cargo), and 9 percent triglycerides (cargo). It binds mainly with cholesterol that has been manufactured by the liver and transports it from the liver to cells.

Lipases: Enzymes (biochemical tools) able to decompose triglycerides (fats).

Lipid: Fat.

Lipoprotein: Lipoproteins are spherical particles consisting of a globule of lipid (fat) molecules surrounded by a protein shell. Lipoproteins are transporter proteins supplying all cells, tissues and organs with fatty acids and cholesterol.

Lipoprotein(a): Lipoprotein(a) is a lipoprotein with two protein shells and one lipid 'core', very similar in lipid composition to LDL, consisting mainly of cholesterol. Lipoprotein(a) is a very adhesive particle; "(a)" stands for "adhesive". Lipoprotein(a), not LDL, is the main risk factor for the development of arteriosclerosis and heart disease or stroke. Lipoprotein(a) is mostly abbreviated to Lp(a).

Metabolic: Of or having to do with metabolism.

Metabolism: The biochemical processes in living organisms that change food into energy, build materials for growth or maintenance, and break down waste products.

Mineral: Minerals are sodium, potassium, magnesium, calcium, chlorine, phosphorus.

Mitochondria: The power stations inside the cells producing cellular energy.

Molecule: The smallest particle into which a substance can be divided without chemical change.

Moribund: Being in the state of dying, approaching death.

Mortality: Death rate.

Myocardial infarction: Interruption of blood supply and heart attack.

Nanogram: 1 nanogram = 1 billionth of a gram.

Nitric oxide: A gas consisting of nitrogen and oxygen used in the body to relax arterial walls.

Nutrient: A nourishing substance, especially as an element or ingredient of a foodstuff.

Organ: Any part of an animal or plant that is composed of various tissues organized to do certain things in the organism. The eyes, heart, kidneys, liver, lungs, etc. are organs of the body.

Organelle: A minute specialized part of a cell, analogous in function to an organ of higher animals.

Organism: A living body having organs that work together to carry on the processes of life; individual plant or animal.

Oxidative: Of or having to do with the action of oxygen.

Oxygen: A gas without color, odor, or taste that forms about one fifth of the air and that is essential for breathing. It is necessary for combustion and for biochemical generation of energy. Oxygen can also be very poisonous. It can damage or destroy vital structures, such as cell walls and artery walls, if there are not enough protecting substances (vitamin C, vitamin E, etc.) present in the body. This situation is comparable to a car: If there were no oxygen, it would never rust, but it would also never run.

Pathological conditions: Diseased conditions, diseases.

Peripheral vascular disease: Arteriosclerosis and subsequent circulatory problems in the legs, kidneys, eyes, etc.

Permeability: Micro-porosity of the capillary walls to provide a passage for nutrients.

Physical: Of or having to do with the body.

Platelet: A very small blood cell, shaped like a disc. Platelets help to clot the blood in order to stop a bleeding.

Platelet aggregation: Clotting of platelets.

Premortal: Occurring just before death.

Primate: Any of the highest order of mammals, including human beings, apes, monkeys, and lemurs.

Prognosis: Forecast of the probable course of a disease.

Protein: A large molecule made up of a string of connected amino acids.

Renal: Of or having to do with the kidneys.

Smooth muscle cells: A special kind of muscle cells found, for example, in the walls of the intestines or in the walls of the arteries.

Stenosis: A narrowed part of a blood vessel.

Stroke: A sudden, serious illness that occurs when an artery supplying blood to the brain is blocked or bursts, leading to a loss of mobility or the ability to speak clearly, or to death.

Structural formula: Chemical formula showing not only the components, but also the three-dimensional form of a molecule.

Symptom: Sign or indication.

Syndrome: A set of symptoms.

Synthesis: A chemical or biochemical manufacturing. The formation of a compound by the chemical union of simpler compounds, for example, the formation of a protein by the chemical union of amino acids.

Synthesize: To manufacture chemically or biochemically.

Systolic blood pressure: Pressure peak in the arteries caused by a contraction of the heart.

Tissue: A group of similar cells, united to perform a specific function, e.g. muscle tissue. Many tissues contain also fibers.

Tomography: X-ray photography of a structure in a certain layer of tissue in the body.

Trace element: Chemical elements like chromium, selenium, or zinc. These elements are indispensable to the body, but are needed only in small amounts (trace amounts).

Triglycerides: The usual form of any nutritional fat, such as that found in butter or sunflower oil.

Vascular: Of or having to do with blood vessels.

Vascular muscle cells: Muscle cells in the walls of the arteries that are able to constrict or relax the arteries, resulting in a smaller or wider inner diameter.

Vasoconstrictoric: Of or having to do with vasoconstriction.

Vasoconstriction: Tightening of the artery wall resulting in a smaller inner diameter of the artery.

Vasodilatative: Of or having to do with vasodilation.

Vasodilation: Relaxation of the artery wall resulting in a wider inner diameter of the artery.

Vein: The blood vessels that return blood from which the oxygen has been unloaded to the heart and to the lungs.

Vitamin: Vitamins are the vital biochemical tools of the body with which the body builds up its structure, including its cells and tissues—muscles, brain, etc.—and with which it breaks down and detoxifies its waste products. Without vitamins, the body would die quickly. The body cannot manufacture vitamins; they have to be absorbed through food and—because the food today is generally depleted—via vitamin supplements.

World Health Organization (WHO): An agency acting within the United Nations.

—— REFERENCES ——

1. Sardi B: Report: What you ought to know about cholesterol-lowering drugs. February 2003.

2. Med World News 1992; March: 27 - 31.

3. Dzugan SA, Arnold Smith R: Hypercholesterolemia treatment: a new hypothesis or just an accident? Med Hypotheses 2002; 59: 751-6

4. Kummerow FA, Olinescu RM, Fleischer L, Handler B, Shinkareva SV: The relationship of oxidized lipids to coronary artery stenosis. Arteriosclerosis 2000; 149: 181-90.

5. Strandberg TE, Salomaa VV, Naukkarinen VA, Vanhanen HT, Sarna SJ, Miettinen TA: Long-term mortality after 5-year multifactorial primary prevention of cardiovascular diseases in middle-aged men. JAMA 1991; 266: 1225-1229.

6. Behar S, Graff E, Reicher-Reiss H, et al: Low total cholesterol is associated with high total mortality in patients with coronary heart disease. The Bezafibrate Infarction Prevention (BIP) Study Group. Eur Heart J 1997; 18: 52-59.

7. Kim JM, Stewart R, Shin IS, Yoon JS: Low cholesterol, cognitive function and Alzheimer's disease in a community population with cognitive impairment. Journal of Nutrition, Health and Aging 2002; 6: 320-323.

8. Kaltenbach M: Serumcholesterol und Koronarsklerose. Fortsch Med 1991; 109, 20: 411-414.

9. Kaltenbach M: Ist erhoehtes Cholesterin die Ursache der Arteriosklerose? Versicherungsmedizin 1995; 47, 4: 112-115.

10. Dietl H, Ohlenschlaeger G: Handbuch der orthomolekularen Medizin. Heidelberg: Haug 1994.

11. Taubes G: What If It's All Been a Big Fat Lie? New York Times Magazine, July 7, 2002.

12. Hartenbach W: Die Cholesterin-Lüge. Das Märchen vom bösen Cholesterin. Muenchen: Herbig 2003.

13. Newman TB: Der Nutzen einer Cholesterinsenkung ist ein theoretisches Modell, das von der Praxis nicht bestätigt wird. Iatros Kardiologie 1994; 3, Supplement: 13-15.

14. Ravnskov U: Cholesterol lowering trials in coronary heart disease: frequency of citation and outcome. BMJ 1992; 305: 15-19.

15. Graveline D: Lipitor® - Thief of Memory - Statin Drugs and the Misguided War On Cholesterol. Haverford: Infinity Publishing 2004.

16. Hartenbach W: Cholesterin - wertvollster Baustein des Lebens. Berlin: Frieling 1999.

17. Skrabanek P: Eine Cholesterinsenkung hat keine Wirkung auf die Gesamt-sterblichkeit. Iatros Kardiologie 1994; 3, Supplement: 16-19.]

18. Rath M: Warum bekommen Tiere keine Herzinfarkt - aber wir Menschen. (Title of the English edition: Why animals don't get heart attack - but people do!) Almelo: MR Publishing 1998.

19. Newman TB, Hulley SB: Cancerogenicity of lipid-lowering drugs. Journal of the American Medical Association 1996; 275: 55-60.

20. Walli AK: Cholesterol and cancer. May Symposium on lipids and lipoproteins. Sponsored by MSD Sharp & Dohme at al. University Hospital Grosshadern, Munich, May 1998.

21. Chang AK, Barrett-Connor E, Edelstein S: Low plasma cholesterol predicts an increased risk of lung cancer in elderly women. Prev Med 1995; 24: 557-562.

22. Voet D, Voet JG: Biochemie. Weinheim, New York, Basel, Cambridge, Tokyo: VCH 1994.

23. Junqueira LC, Carneiro J, Kelley RO: Histologie. Berlin, Heidelberg, New York, Barcelona, Hongkong, London, Milan, Paris, Tokyo: Springer 2002.

24. Gröber U: Orthomolekulare Medizin - ein Leitfaden fuer Apotheker und Aerzte. Stuttgart: Wissenschaftliche Verlagsgesellschaft 2002.

25. Langsjoen PH: The clinical use of HMG CoA-reductase inhibitors (statins) and the associated depletion of the essential co-factor coenzyme Q10; a review of pertinent human and animal data. http://www.fda.gov/ohrms/dockets/dailys/02/May02/052902/02p-0244-cp00001-02-Exhibit_A-vol1.pdf.

26. Papers from the Third Conference of the International Coenzyme Q10 Association. London, United Kingdom. November 22-24, 2002. Biofactors 2003; 18(1-4): 1-314.

27. Langsjoen PH: Statin-induced cardiomyopathy. Introduction to the citizen's petition on statins. http://www.redflagsweekly.com/features/2002_july08P.html.

27A. Rizvi K, Hampson JP, Harvey JN: Do lipid-lowering drugs cause erectile dysfunction? A systematic review. Family Practice 2002; 19: 95-98.

27B. Solomon H, Samarasinghe YP, Feher MD, Man J, Rivas-Toro H, Lumb PJ, Wierzbicki AS, Jackson G: Erectile dysfunction and statin treatment in high cardiovascular risk patients. Int J Clin Pract 2006; 60(2): 141-145.

28. Edison RJ, Muenke M: Central nervous system and limb anomalies in case reports of first-trimester statin exposure. N Engl J Med 2004; 350:1579-1582.

29. Psychoneuroendocrinology 2003; 28: 181-194.

30. Minerva Med 1995; 86: 251-256.

31. J Behav Med 1996; 22: 82-84.

32. Zureik M, Courbon D, Ducimetiere P: Serum cholesterol concentration and death from suicide in men: Paris prospective study I. BMJ 1996; 313: 649-651.

33. Mufti RM, Balon R, Arfken CL: Low Cholesterol and Violence. Psychiatr Serv 1998; 49: 221-224.

34. Golomb BA: Cholesterol and violence: is there a connection? Ann Intern Med 1998; 128: 478-487.

35. Borgers D: Cholesterin: Das Scheitern eines Dogmas. Berlin: Edition Sigma 1993.

36. Bruker MO, Gutjahr I: Cholesterin - der lebensnotwendige Stoff. Lahnstein: Emu 2002.

37. Garland CF, Garland FC, Gorham ED, Lipkin M, Newmark H, Mohr SB, Holick MF: The Role of Vitamin D in Cancer Prevention. Am J Public Health 2006; 96: 9-18.

38. Löffler G, Petrides PE: Biochemie und Pathobiochemie. Berlin, Heidelberg, New York: Springer 2003.

38A. Ravnskov U: High cholesterol may protect against infections and atherosclerosis. Q J Med 2003; 96: 927-934.

39. Ginter E: Vitamin C deficiency, cholesterol metabolism and arteriosclerosis. J Orthomol Med 1991; 6; 166.

40. Sokoloff B, Hori M, Saelhof CC, Wrzolek T, Imai T: Aging, arteriosclerosis and ascorbic acid metabolism. Journal of the American Geriatric Society 1966; 14: 1239-1260.

41. Ginter E: Cholesterol: Vitamin C controls its transformation into bile acids. Science 1973; 179: 702.

42. Ginter E: Marginal vitamin C deficiency, lipid metabolism, and arteriosclerosis. Lipid Research 1978; 16: 216-220.

43. Harwood HJ Jr, Greene YJ, Stacpoole PW: Inhibition of human leucocyte 3-hydroxy-3-methylglutaryl coenzyme A reductase activity by ascorbic acid. An effect mediated by the free radical monodehydro-vitamin C. J Biol Chem 1986; 261: 7127-7135.

44. Hemilä H: Vitamin C and blood cholesterol. In: Critical Reviews in Food Science and Nutrition 1986; 32 (1): 33-57, CRC Press Inc., Florida.

45. Alderman JD, et al: Effect of a modified, well-tolerated niacin regimen on serum total cholesterol, high density lipoprotein cholesterol and the cholesterol to high density lipoprotein ratio. Am J Cardiol 1989; 64: 725-29.

46. Altschul R, Hoffer A, Stephen JD: Influence of nicotinic acid on serum cholesterol in man. Arch Biochem Biophys 1955; 54: 558-559.

47. Carlson LA, Hamsten A, Asplund A: Pronounced lowering of serum levels of lipoprotein Lp(a) in hyperlipidemic subjects treated with nicotinic acid. J Inter Med 1989; 226: 271-276.

48. Parsons WB Jr, Achor RWP, Berge KG, McKenzie BF, Barker NW: Changes in concentration of blood lipids following prolonged administration of nicotinic acid to persons with hypercholesterolemia: prelimary observations. Proc Mayo Clinic 1956; 31: 377-390.

49. Guraker A, Hoeg JM, Kostner G, Papadopoulos NM, Brewer HB Jr: Levels of lipoprotein Lp(a) decline with neomycin and niacin treatment. Arteriosclerosis 1985; 57: 293-301.

50. Lavie CJ: Marked benefit with sustained-release niacin (vitamin B3) therapy in patients with isolated very low levels of high-density lipoprotein cholesterol and coronary artery disease. Am J Cardiol 1992; 69: 1093-1085.

51. Avogaro P, Bon GB, Fusello M: Effect of pantethine on lipids, lipoproteins and apolipoproteins in man. Curr Ther Res 1983; 33: 488-493.

52. Gaddi A, Descovich GC, Noseda G, Fragiacomo C, Colombo L, Craveri A, Montanari G, Sirtori CR: Controlled evaluation of pantethine, a natural hypolipidemic compound, in patients with different forms of hyperlipoproteinemia. Arteriosclerosis 1984; 5: 73-83.

53. Hermann WJ Jr, Ward K, Faucett J: The effect of tocopherol on high-density lipoprotein cholesterol. A clinical observation. Am J Clin Pathol 1979; 72: 848-852.

54. Beamish R: Vitamin E - then and now. Can J Cardiol 1993; 9: 29-31.

55. Opie LH: Review: Role of carnitine in fatty acid metabolism of normal and ischemic myocardium. Am Heart J 1979; 97: 375-388.

56. Cherchi A, Lai C, Angelino F, Trucco G, Caponnetto S, Mereto PE, Rosolen G, Manzoli U, Schiavoni G, Reale A, et al: Effects of L-carnitine on exercise tolerance in chronic stable angina: a multicenter, double-blind, randomized, placebo-controlled crossover study. Int J Clin Pharmacol Ther Toxicol 1985; 23(10): 569-572.

57. Khan A, Safdar M, Khan MMA, Khattak KN, Anderson RA: Cinnamon improves glucose and lipids of people with type 2 diabetes. Diabetes Care 2003; 26: 3215-3218.

58. Anderson JW, Jones AE, Riddell-Mason S: Ten different dietary fibers have significantly different effects on serum and liver lipids of cholesterol-fed rats. J Nutr 1994; 124: 78-83.

59. Avivi-Green C, Polak-Charcon S, Madar Z, Schwartz B: Dietary regulation and localization of apoptosis cascade proteins in the colonic crypt. J Cell Biochem 2000; 77: 18-29.

60. Cerda JJ, Normann SJ, Sullivan MP, et al: Inhibition of arteriosclerosis by dietary pectin in microswine with sustained hypercholesterolemia. Circulation 1994; 89: 1247-1253.

61. Cerda JJ, Robbins FL, Burgin CW, et al: The effects of grapefruit pectin on patients at risk for coronary heart disease without altering diet or lifestyle. Clin Cardiol 1988; 11: 589-594.

62. Ebihara K, Kiriyama S, Manabe M: Cholesterol-lowering activity of various natural pectins and synthetic pectin-derivatives with different physico-chemical properties. Nutr Rep Int 1979; 20: 519-526.

63. Ginter E, Kubec FJ, Vozar J, et al: Natural hypocholesterolemic agent: pectin plus ascorbic acid. Int J Vitam Nutr Res (Switzerland) 1979; 49(4): 406-412.

64. Hillman LC, Peters SG, Fisher CA, Pomare EW: The effects of the fiber components pectin, cellulose and lignin on serum cholesterol levels. Am J Clin Nutr 1985; 42: 207-213.

65. Judd PA, Truswell AS: The hypocholesterolemic effects of pectins in rats. Br J Nutr 1985; 53: 409-425.

66. Kay RM, Truswell AS: Effects of citrus pectin on blood lipids and fecal steroid excretion in man. Am J Clin Nutr 1977; 30: 171-175.

67. Platt D, Raz A: Modulation of the lung colonization of B16-F1 melanoma cells by citrus pectin. J Natl Cancer Inst 1992; 84: 438-442.

68. Richter WO, Jacob BG, Schwandt P: Interaction between fibre and lovastatin. Lancet 1991; 338: 706.

69. Riedl J, Linseisen J, Hoffman J, Wolfran G: Some dietary fibers reduce the absorption of carotenoids in women. J Nutr 1999; 129: 2170-2176.

70. Rock CL, Swendseid ME: Blood beta-carotene response in humans after meals supplemented with dietary pectin. Am J Clin Nutr 1992; 55: 96-99.

71. Terpstra AHM, Lapre JA, de Vries HT, Beynen AC: Dietary pectin with high viscosity lowers blood and liver cholesterol concentration and blood ester transfer protein activity in hamsters. J Nutr 1998; 128: 1944-1949.

72. Veldman FJ, Nair CH, Vorster HH, et al: Possible mechanism through which dietary pectin influences fibrin network architecture in hypercholesterolaemic subjects. Thromb Res 1999; 93: 253-264.

73. World Health Organization, http://www.who.int/cardiovascular_diseases/en.

74. Rath M, Pauling L: Hypothesis: Lipoprotein(a) is a surrogate for vitamin C. Proc Natl Acad Sci USA 1990; 87, 6204-6207.

75. Rath M, Pauling L: Solution of the puzzle of human cardiovascular disease: Its primary cause is vitamin C deficiency, leading to the deposition of lipoprotein(a) and fibrinogen/fibrin in the vascular wall. J Orthomol Med 1991; 6: 125-134.

76. Rath M: Reducing the risk for cardiovascular disease with nutritional supplements. J Orthomol Med 1992; 7, 153-162.

77. Buddecke E: Grundriss der Biochemie. Berlin, New York: De Gruyter 1994.

78. Schnare DW, Denk G, Shields M, Brunton S: Evaluation of a detoxification regimen for fat stored xenobiotics. Medical Hypotheses 1982; 9: 265-282.

79. Pauling L: How to live longer and feel better. New York: W. H. Freeman 1985.

80. Brubacher G et al.: Vitamine und Krebsprävention. Vitaminspur 1987; 2:188-192.

81. Waldeyer A: Anatomie des Menschen. Berlin, New York: De Gruyter 1974.

82. Chowka PB: Linus Pauling, The Last Interview. http://members.aol.com/realmedia/pauling.html.

83. Zuckerkandl E, Pauling L: Molecular disease, evolution, and genic heterogeneity. In: Horizons on Biochemistry, eds. Kasha M, Pullman B. New York: Academic Press 1962; 189-225.

84. Nishikimi M, Udenfriend S: Immunologic evidence that the gene for L-gulono-gamma-lactone oxidase is not expressed in animals subject to scurvy. Proc Nat Acad Sci 1976; 73: 2066-2068.

85. Nishikimi M, Koshizaka T, Ozawa T, Yagi K: Occurrence in humans and guinea pigs of the gene related to their missing enzyme L-gulono-gamma-lactone oxidase. Arch Biochem Biophys 1988; 267: 842-846.

86. Nishikimi M, Kawai T, Yagi K: Guinea pigs possess a highly mutated gene for L-gulono-gamma-lactone oxidase, the key enzyme for L-ascorbic acid biosynthesis missing in this species. J Biol Chem 1992; 267: 21967-21972.

87. Rath M, Pauling L: A unified theory of human cardiovascular disease leading the way to the abolition of this disease as a cause for human mortality. J Orthomol Med 1992: 7: 5-15.

88. Kawai T, Nishikimi M, Ozawa T, Yagi K: A missense mutation of L-gulono-gamma-lactone oxidase causes the inability of scurvy-prone osteogenic disorder rats to synthesize L-ascorbic acid. J Biol Chem 1992; 267: 21973-21976.

89. Nishikimi M, Fukuyama R, Minoshima S, Shimizu N, Yagi K: Cloning and chromosomal mapping of the human nonfunctional gene for L-gulono-gamma-lactone oxidase, the enzyme for L-ascorbic acid biosynthesis missing in man. J Biol Chem 1994; 269: 13685-13688.

90. Stryer L: Biochemistry. New York: W. H. Freeman 1995.

91. Cameron E, Pauling L, Leibovitz B: Ascorbic acid and cancer: a review. Cancer Research 1979; 39: 663-681.

92. Rath M, Pauling L: Apoprotein(a) is an adhesive protein. J Orthomol Med 1991; 6: 139-143.

93. Gaubatz JW, Heideman C, Gotto AM, Morrisett JD, Dahlen GH: Human blood lipoprotein(a): structural properties. J Biol Chem 1983; 258: 4582-4589.

94. Utermann G, Weber W: Protein composition of Lp(a) lipoprotein from human blood. FEBS Lett 1983; 154: 357-361.

95. Rath M, Niendorf A, Reblin T, Dietel M, Krebber HJ, Beisiegel U: Detection and quantification of lipoprotein (a) in the arterial wall of 107 coronary bypass patients. Arteriosclerosis 1989; 9: 579-592.

96. Beisiegel U, Niendorf A, Wolf K, Reblin T, Rath M: Lipoprotein (a) in the arterial wall. European Heart Journal 1990; 11: Suppl. E, 174-183.

97. Miles LA, Fless GM, Levin EG, Scanu AM, Plow EF: A potential basis for the thrombotic risk associated with lipoprotein(a). Nature 1989; 339: 301-302.

98. Hajjar KA, Gavish D, Breslow JL, Nachmann RL: Lipoprotein(a) modulation of endothelial cell surface fibrinolysis and its potential role in arteriosclerosis. Nature 1989; 339: 303-305.

99. Harpel PC, Gordon BR, Parker TS: Plasmin catalyzes binding of lipoprotein(a) to immobilized fibrinogen and fibrin. Proc Natl Acad Sci USA 1989; 86, 3847-3851.

100. Niendorf A, Rath M, Wolf K, Peters S, Arps H, Beisiegel U, Dietel M: Morphological detection and quantification of lipoprotein(a) deposition in atheromatous lesions of human aorta and coronary arteries. Virchow's Archiv A Pathol Anat 1990; 417: 105-111.

101. Karadi I, Kostner GM, Gries A, Nimpf J, Romics L, Malle E: Lipoprotein(a) and plasminogen are immunochemically related. Biochimica et Biophysica Acta 1988; 960: 91-97.

102. Knox EG: Ischaemic-heart-disease mortality and dietary intake of calcium. The Lancet 1973; 1: 1465-1467.

103. Armstrong VW, Cremer P, Egerle E, Manke A, Schulze F, Wieland H, Kreuzer H, Seidel D: The association between serum Lp(a) concentrations and angiographically assessed coronary arteriosclerosis: dependence on serum LDL levels. Arteriosclerosis 1986; 62: 249-257.

104. Dahlen GH, Guyton JR, Attar M, Farmer JA, Kautz JA, Gotto AM Jr.: Association of levels of lipoprotein Lp(a), blood lipids, and other lipoproteins with coronary artery disease documented by angiography. Circulation 1986; 74: 758-765.

104A. Kamstrup PR, Tybjaerg-Hansen A, Steffensen R, Nordestgaard BG: Genetically elevated lipoprotein(a) and increased risk of myocardial infarction. JAMA 2009; 301(22): 2331-2339.

105. Zenker G, Koltringer P, Bone G, Kiederkorn K, Pfeiffer K, Jurgens G: Lipoprotein(a) as a strong indicator for cerebrovascular disease. Stroke 1986; 17: 942-945.

106. Jürgens G, Taddei-Peters WC, Költringer P, Petek W, Chen Q, Greilberger J, Macomber PF, Butman BT, Stead AG, Ransom JH: Lipoprotein(a) serum cooncentration and apolipoprotein(a) phenotype correlate with severity and presence of ischemic cerebrovascular disease. Stroke 1995; 26: 1841-1848.

107. Hoff HF, Gaubatz JW: Isolation, purification, and characterization of a lipoprotein containing apo B from human aorta. Arteriosclerosis 1982; 42: 273-297.

108. Kostner GM, Avogaro P, Cazzolato G, Marth E, Bittolo-Bon G, Qunici GB: Lipoprotein Lp(a) and the risk for myocardial infarction. Arteriosclerosis 1981; 38: 51-61.

109. Kostner GM, Gavish D, Leopold B, Bolzano K, Weintraub MS, Breslow JL: HMG CoA reductase inhibitors lower LDL cholesterol without reducing Lp(a) levels. Circulation 1989; 80: 1313-1319.

110. Lawn RM: Lipoprotein(a) in heart disease. Scientific American 1992; 266, 6: 54-60.

111. Pauling L: Vitamin C and cardiovascular disease. Medical Science Research 1991; 19: 398.

112. Rath M, Pauling L: An orthomolecular theory of human health and disease. J Orthomol Med 1991; 6: 135-138.

113. Gey FK, Staehelin HB, Eichholzer M: Poor blood status of carotene and vitamin C is associated with a higher mortality from ischemic heart disease and stroke: Basel Prospective Study. Clin Invest 1993; 71: 3-6.

114. Gey FK: Ten-year retrospective on the antioxidant hypothesis of arteriosclerosis: threshold blood levels of antioxidant micronutrients related to minimum cardiovascular risk. J Nutr Biochem 1995; 6:206-36

115. Canner PL, Berge KG, Wenger NK, Stamler J, Friedman L, Prineas RJ, Friedewald W: Fifteen year mortality in Coronary Drug Project patients: long-term benefit with niacin. J Am Coll Cardiol. 1986; 8: 1245-1255.

116. Hoffer A: Niacin, coronary disease and longevity. J Orthomol Med 1989; 4: 211-220.

117. Singh RB, Niaz MA: Serum concentration of lipoprotein(a) decreases on treatment with hydrosoluble coenzyme Q10 in patients with coronary artery disease: discovery of a new role. Int J Cardiol 1999; 68 :23-9.

118. Herrmann W et al.: Beeinflussung des atherogenen Risikofaktors Lp(a) durch supplementaere Fischoelaufnahme bei Patienten mit moderatem physischem Training. Medizinische Klinik 1989; 84: 429-433.

119. Gavish D, Breslow JL: Lipoprotein(a) reduction by N-acetylcysteine. Lancet 1991; 337: 203-204.

120. Beetens JR, Coene MC, Veheyen A, Zonnekeyn L, Herman AG: Vitamin C increases the prostacyclin production and decreases the vascular lesions in experimental arteriosclerosis in rabbits. Prostaglandins 1986; 32: 335-352.

121. Williams RJ: Nutrition against disease. New York: Pitman 1971.

122. Rath M, Pauling L: Immunological evidence for the accumulation of lipoprotein(a) in the arteriosclerotic lesion of the hypoascorbemic guinea pig. Proc Natl Acad Sci USA 1990; 87, 9388-9390.

123. Simon JA, Murtaugh MA, Gross MD, Loria CM, Hulley SB, Jacobs DR: Relation of ascorbic acid to coronary artery calcium. American Journal of Epidemiology 2004; 159: 581-588

124. Ginter E: Chronic marginal vitamin C deficiency: biochemistry and pathophysiology. World Rev Nutr Diet 1979; 33: 104-141.

125. Bates CJ, Mandal AR, Cole TJ: HDL cholesterol and vitamin C status. Lancet 1977; II: 611.

126. Jialal I, Vega GL, Grundy SM: Physiologic levels of vitamin C inhibit the oxidative modification of low density lipoprotein. Arteriosclerosis 1990; 82: 185-191.

127. Brody S: High-dose ascorbic acid increases intercourse frequency and improves mood: a randomized controlled clinical trial. Biological Psychiatry 2002; 52: 371-374.

128. Hickey S, Roberts H: Ascorbate. The Science of Vitamin C. ISBN 1-4116-0724-4.

129. Enstrom JE, Kanim LE, Klein MA: Vitamin C intake and mortality among a sample of the United States population. Epidemiology 1992; 3: 194-202.

130. Bolton-Smith C, Woodward M, Tunstall-Pedoe H: The Scottish Heart Health Study. Dietary intake by food frequency questionnaire and odds ratios for coronary heart disease risk. II. The antioxidant vitamins and fibre. Eur J Clin Nutr 1992; 46: 85-93.

131. Yokoyama T, Chigusa D, Kokubo Y, Yoshiike N, Matsumura Y, Tanaka H: Serum vitamin C concentration was inversely associated with subsequent 20-year incidence of stroke in a Japanese rural community. Stroke 2000;31:2287-2294.

132. Nyyssönen K, Parviainen MT, Salonen R, Tuomilehto J, Salonen JT: Vitamin C deficiency and risk of myocardial infarction: prospective population study of men from eastern Finland. BMJ 1997; 314: 634-638.

132A. Simon JA, Hudes ES, Browner WS: Serum ascorbic acid and cardiovascular disease prevalence in U.S. adults. Epidemiology 1998; 9(3): 316-321.

133. Rimm EB, Stampfer MJ, Ascherio A, Giovannucci E, Colditz GA, Willett WC: Vitamin E consumption and the risk of coronary heart disease in men. New Engl J Med 1993; 328: 1450-1456.

134. Stampfer MJ, Hennekens CH, Manson JE, Colditz GA, Rosner B, Willett WC: Vitamin E consumption and the risk of coronary heart disease in women. New Engl J Med 1993; 328: 1444-1449.

135. Gey KF, Puska P, Jordan P, Moser UK: Inverse correlation between plasma vitamin E and mortality from ischemic heart disease in cross-cultural epidemiology. Am J Clin Nutr 1991; 53: 326S-334S.

136. Jackson ML: Selenium: geochemical distribution and associations with human heart and cancer death rates and longevity in China and the United States. Biol Trace Elem Res 1988; 15: 13-21.

137. Schmidt K, Bayer W: Selen - Aktueller wissenschaftlicher Erkenntnisstand. VitaMinSpur 1988; 3: Suppl. 1, 1-20.

138. Ubbink JB, Vermaak WJ, van der Merwe A, Becker PJ: Vitamin B12, vitamin B6 and folate nutritional status in men with hyperhomocysteinemia. Am J Clin Nutr 1993; 57: 47-53.

139. Ovebro KK, Svardal A: The effect of glutathione modulation on the concentration of homocysteine in plasma of rats. Pharmacol Toxicol 2000; 87, 103-107.

140. Wiklund O, Fager G, Andersson A, Lundstam U, Masson P, Hultberg B: N-acetylcysteine treatment lowers plasma homocysteine but not serum lipoprotein(a) levels. Atherosclerosis 1996; 119, 99-106.

141. Ventura P, Panini R, Pasini MC, Scarpetta G, Salvioli G: N-Acetylcysteine reduces homocysteine plasma levels after single intravenous administration by increasing thiols urinary excretion. Pharmacol Res 1999; 40, 345-350.

142. Paterson JC: Some factors in the causation of intimal hemorrhages and in the precipitation of coronary thrombi. Canadian Medical Association Journal 1941; 44: 114-120.

143. Willis GC, Light AW, Gow WQS: Serial arteriography in arteriosclerosis. Can Med Assoc J 1954; 71: 562-568.

144. Willis GC: The Reversibility of Arteriosclerosis. Can Med Assoc J 1957; 77: 106-109.

145. Stone I: The genetic disease hypoascorbemia. Acta Geneticae Medicae et Gemellologicae 1967; 16: 52-60.

146. Committee on Animal Nutrition: Nutrient Requirements for Laboratory Animals, Pub. No. 990, National Academy of Science.

147. Stolman JM, Goldman HM, Gould BS: Ascorbic acid in blood vessels. Arch Pathol 1961; 72: 59-68.

148. Rath M, Niedzwiecki A: Nutritional supplement program halts progression of early coronary arteriosclerosis documented by ultrafast computed tomography. Journal of Applied Nutrition 1996; 48: 68-78.

149. Mead C, Hager T: Linus Pauling: Scientist and Peacemaker. Corvallis: Oregon State University Press 2001.

150. Riemersma RA, Wood DA, MacIntyre CCA, Elton RA, Gey KF, Oliver MF: Risk of angina pectoris and blood concentrations of vitamin A, C, and E and carotene. Lancet 1991; 337: 1-5.

151. Hodis HN, Mack WJ, LaBree L, et al: Serial coronary angiographic evidence that antioxidant vitamin intake reduces progression of coronary artery arteriosclerosis. JAMA.1995; 273: 1849-1854.

152. Morrison HI, Schaubel D, Desmeules M, Wigle DT: Serum folate and risk of fatal coronary heart disease. JAMA 1996; 275:1893-1896.

153. Egashira K, Hirooka Y, Kuga T, Mohri M, Takeshita A: Effects of L-arginine supplementation on endothelium-dependent coronary vasodilation in patients with angina pectoris and normal coronary arteriograms. Circulation 1996; 92: 130-134.

154. Tousoulis D, Davies G, Tentolouris C, Crake T, Toutouzas P: Coronary stenosis dilatation induced by L-arginine. Lancet 1997; 349: 1812-1813.

155. Clarkson P, Adams MR, Powe AJ, Donald AE, McCredie R, Robinson J, McCarthy SN, Keech A, Celermajer DS, Deanfield JE: Oral L-arginine improves endothelium-dependent dilatation in hypercholesterolemic young adults. J Clin Invest 1996; 97: 1989-1994.

156. Wolf A, Zalpour C, Theilmeier G, Wang BY, Ma A, Anderson B, Tsao PS, Cooke JP: Dietary L-arginine supplementation normalizes platelet aggregation in hypercholesterolemic humans. J Am Coll Cardiol 1997; 29: 479-485.

157. Ceremuzynski L, Chamiec T, Herbaczynska-Cedro K.: Effect of supplemental oral L-arginine on exercise capacity in patients with stable angina pectoris. Am J Cardiol 1997; 80: 331-333.

158. Rath M, Pauling L: Case report: Lysine/vitamin C-related amelioration of angina pectoris. J Orthomol Med 1991; 6: 144-146.

159. Rath M: Lipoprotein(a) reduction by vitamin C. Journal of Orthomolecular Medicine 1992; 7: 81-82.

160. McBeath M, Pauling L: A case history: Lysine/vitamin C-related amelioration of angina pectoris. Journal of Orthomolecular Medicine 1993; 8, 77-78.

161. Ely JTA: On the Reversal and Prevention of Heart Disease. Seattle: University of Washington 2002.

162. Arbeitskreis Ernährungs- und Vitamin-Information e.V. (evi): Vitamine in Rauch aufgelöst. Fachinformation Vitamine 1986-87; 4.

163. Lee WH: Coenzyme Q10 - is it our new fountain of youth? New Canaan: Keats 1987.

164. Gross R, Kaufmann W, Hilger HH: Innere Medizin. Köln: Herold (Editor), University of Köln 1979.

165. Visioli F, Smith A, Zhang W, Keaney JF Jr, Hagen T, Frei B: Lipoic acid and vitamin C potentiate nitric oxide synthesis in human aortic endothelial cells independently of cellular glutathione status. Redox Rep. 2002; 7: 223-227.

166. Koh ET: Effect of vitamin C on blood parameters of hypertensive subjects. J Oklahoma State Med Assoc 1984; 77: 177-182.

167. Korbut R: Effect of L-arginine on plasminogen activator inhibitor in hypertensive patients with hypercholesterinemia. New England J Med 1993; 328: 287-288.

168. Anabolism J Preventive Med 1983; 2(6): 1.

169. Altura BM, Altura BT: Interactions of Mg and K on blood vessels: Aspects in view of hypertension. Magnesium 1984; 3(4-6): 175-194.

170. Altura BM, Altura BT: Magnesium ions and contraction of vascular smooth muscles: Relationship to some vascular diseases. Fed Proc 1981; 40(12): 2672-2679.

171. Völger KD, Mutschler E: Magnesium - ein überschätztes oder unterbewertetes Pharmakon? Deutsche Apotheker Zeitung 1991; 13: 589-598.

172. Heilmeyer L, Holtmeier HJ: Ernaehrungswissenschaften. Stuttgart: Thieme 1968.

173. Holtmeier HJ: Magnesium-Mangel-Syndrom. Stuttgart: Hippokrates 1988.

174. Wester PO, Dyckner T: The importance of the magnesium ion. Magnesium deficiency - symptomatology and occurrence. Acta Med Scand 1982; 661 (Suppl): 3-4.

175. Dyckner T, Wester PO: Magnesium deficiency - guidelines for diagnosis and substitution therapy. Acta Med Scand 1982; 661 (Suppl): 37-41.

176. Stein-Hammer C: Magnesium in der Naturheilkunde. Erfahrungsheilkunde 1993; 10: 480-486.

177. Seeger PG: Magnesium - ein unentbehrlicher Mineralstoff. Sanum-Post 1990; 13: 14-16.

178. Yeh JK et al.: J Nutr 1986; 116: 273-280.

179. Durlach J: Le Diabete 1971; 19: 99-113.

180. Lindeman RD et al: Magnesium in Health and Disease. Jamaica, N.Y.: S. P. Medical and Scientific Books 1980; 236-245.

181. Abrams KJ, Ludwig H: ADHD - Aufmerksamkeitsstoerung und Hyperaktivitaet bei Kindern und Erwachsenen - Alternativen zur medikamentoesen Behandlung. Neusiedl am See: AV Publication 2000.

182. Bukowski R, Lucas P, Drueke T, McCarron D: Theoretical mechanisms of dietary calcium's antihypertensive action. Adv Exp Med Biol 1986; 208: 389–96.

183. Mikami H, Ogihara T, Tabuchi Y: Blood pressure response to dietary calcium intervention in humans. Am J Hypertens 1990; 3 (Suppl): 147-151.

184. Gillman MW, Belanger A, D'Agostino RB, Ellison RC, Posner BM: Protective effect of calcium intake on development of hypertension. Circulation 1994; 89: 941.

185. Gassmann B, Schultz M, Leist M, Brigelius-Flohé R: Vitamin-E-Stoffwechsel und Bedarf. Ernährungs-Umschau 1995; 42 (3): 80-87.

186. Kamal-Eldin A, Appelqvist LÅ: The chemistry and antioxidant properties of tocopherols and tocotrienols. Lipids 1996; 31: 671-701.

187. Bässler KH, Grün E, Loew D, Pietrzik K: Vitamin-Lexikon für Ärzte, Apotheker und Ernährungswissenschaftler. Stuttgart, Jena, New York: Gustav Fischer 1992.

188. Ohlenschläger G: Das Vitaminoid: Ubichinon (Coenzym Q10). J Orthomolekulare Medizin 1994; 3.

189. Yamamura Y, Ishiyama T, Yamagomai T, et al: Clinical use of coenzyme Q for treatment of cardiovascular disease. Jpn Circ J 1967; 31: 168.

190. Iwamoto Y, Yamagami T, Folkers K, et al: Deficiency of coenzyme Q10 in hypertensive rats and reduction of deficiency by treatment with coenzyme Q10. Biochem Biophys Res Commun 1974; 58: 743-748.

191. Yamagami T, Shibata N, Folkers K: Bioenergetics in clinical medicine. Studies on coenzyme Q10 and essential hypertension. Res Commun Chem Pathol Pharmacol 1975; 11: 273-288.

192. Yamagami T, Shibata N, Folkers K: Bioenergetics in clinical medicine. VIII. Administration of coenzyme Q10 to patients with essential hypertension. Res Commun Chem Pathol Pharmacol 1976; 14: 721-727.

193. Folkers K, Drzewoski J, Richardson PC, et al: Bioenergetics in clinical medicine. XVI. Reduction of hypertension in patients by therapy with coenzyme Q10. Res Commun Chem Pathol Pharmacol 1981; 31: 129-140.

194. Yamagami T, Takagi M, Akagami H, et al: Effect of coenzyme Q10 on essential hypertension: a double-blind controlled study. Biomedical and clinical aspects of coenzyme Q. Folkers K (ed). Amsterdam, Elsevier Science Publications 1986; 5: 337-343.

195. Digiesi V, Cantini F, Brodbeck B: Effect of coenzyme Q10 on essential arterial hypertension. Curr Ther Res 1990; 47: 841-845.

196. Digiesi V, Cantini F, Bisi G, Guarino GC, Oradei A, Littarru GP: Mechanism of action of coenzyme Q10 in essential hypertension. Curr Ther Res 1992; 51: 668-672.

197. Langsjoen PH, Langjoen P, Willis R, et al.: Treatment of essential hypertension with coenzyme Q10. Mol Aspects Med 1994; 15 (Suppl): 265-272.

198. Singh RB, Niaz MA, Rastogi SS, et al: Effect of hydrosoluble coenzyme Q10 on blood pressures and insulin resistance in hypertensive patients with coronary artery disease. J Hum Hypertens 1999; 13: 203-208.

199. Palumbo G, Avanzini F, Alli C, et al: Effects of vitamin E on clinic and ambulatory blood pressure in treated hypertensive patients. Collaborative group of the Primary Prevention Project (PPP) hypertension study. Am J Hypertens 2000; 13: 564-567.

200. Burke BE, Neuenschwander R, Olson RD: Randomized, double-blind, placebo-controlled trial of coenzyme Q10 in isolated systolic hypertension. South Med J 2001; 94(11): 1112-1117.

201. Barrie SA, Wright JV, Pizzorno JE: Effects of garlic oil on platelet aggregation, serum lipids and blood pressure in humans. J Orthomol Med 1987; 2: 15-21.

202. Wendt L: Krankheiten verminderter Kapillarmembranpermeabilität. Frankfurt: E. E. Koch 1973.

202A. Steffen LM, Kroenke CH, Yu X, Pereira MA, Slattery ML, van Horn L, Gross MD, Jacobs DR Jr: Associations of plant food, dairy product, and meat intakes with 15-y incidence of elevated blood pressure in young black and white adults: the Coronary Artery Risk Development in Young Adults (CARDIA) Study. Am J Clin Nutr 2005; 82(6), 1169-1177.

203. Fonorow OR: Nature's perfect statin. Vitamin C is the original HMG-CoA reductase inhibitor. http://www.thecureforheartdisease.com/owen/alice.htm.

204. Harwood HJ Jr, Greene YJ, Stacpoole PW: Inhibition of human leukocyte 3-hydroxy-3-methylglutaryl coenzyme A reductase activity by ascorbic acid. An effect mediated by the free radical monodehydroascorbate. J Biol Chem 1986; 261: 7127-35.

205. Ehmke J: More reasons to avoid statin drugs. Does Lipitor raise Lp(a)? http://www.mercola.com/2003/aug/13/statin_drugs.htm.

206. Goodman T: Lipoprotein ups heart attack risk. Associated Press National, 4 September 2000.

207. Danesh J, Collins R, Peto R: Lipoprotein(a) and coronary heart disease. Meta-analysis of prospective studies. Circulation 2000; 102: 1082-5.

208. Passi S, Stancato A, Aleo E, Dmitrieva A, Littarru GP: Statins lower plasma and lymphocyte ubiquinol/ubiquinone without affecting other antioxidants and PUFA. Biofactors 2003; 18: 113-124

209. Shimon I, Almog S, Vered Z, Seligmann H, Shefi M, Peleg E, Rosenthal T, Motro M, Halkin H, Ezra D: Improved left ventricular function after thiamine supplementation in patients with congestive heart failure receiving long-term furosemide therapy. Am J Med 1995; 98: 485-490.

210. Yamamura Y, Ishiyama T, Yamagomai T, et al: Clinical use of coenzyme Q for treatment of cardiovascular disease. Jpn Circ J 1967; 31: 168.

211. Folkers K, Vadhanavikit S, Mortensen SA: Biochemical rationale and myocardial tissue data on the effective therapy of cardiomyopathy with coenzyme Q10. Proc Natl Acad Sci USA 1985; 82: 901-904.

212. Langsjoen PH, Vadhanavikit S, Folkers K: Response of patients in classes III and IV of cardiomyopathy to therapy in a blind and crossover trial with coenzyme Q10. Proc Natl Acad Sci USA 1985; 82: 4240-4244.

213. Langsjoen PH, Folkers K, Lyson K, Muratsu K, Lyson T, Langjoen P: Effective and safe therapy with coenzyme Q10 for cardiomyopathy. Klinische Wochenschrift 1988; 66: 583-590.

214. Langsjoen PH, Folkers K, Lyson K, Muratsu K, Lyson T, Langjoen P: Pronounced increase of survival of patients with cardiomyopathy when treated with coenzyme Q10 and conventional therapy. Int J Tissue Reactions 1990; 13: 163-168.

215. Morisco C, Trimarco B, Condorelli M: Effect of coenzyme Q10 in patients with congestive heart failure: a long-term multicenter randomized study. Clin Invest 1993; 71: 134-136.

216. Baggio E, Gandini R, Plancher AC, et al: Italian multicenter study on safety and efficacy of coenzyme Q10 adjunctive therapy in heart failure. Mol Aspects Med 1994; 15 (Suppl): 287-294.

217. Suzuki Y, Masumura Y, Kobayashi A, et al: Myocardial carnitine deficiency in chronic heart failure. Lancet 1982; i; 116.

218. Kobayashi A, Masumara Y, Yamazaki N: L-carnitine treatment for congestive heart failure: experimental and clinical study. Jap Circul J 1992; 56: 86-94.

219. Bartels GL, Remme WJ, Pillay M, et al: Effects of L-propionylcarnitine on ischemia-induced myocardial dysfunction in men with angina pectoris. Am J Cardiol 1994; 74: 125-130.

220. Azuma J, Hasegawa H, Sawamura N, et al: Taurine for treatment of congestive heart failure. Int J Cardiol 1982; 2: 303-304.

221. Rector TS, Bank A, Mullen KA, et al: Randomized, double-blind, placebo controlled study of supplemental oral L-arginine in patients with heart failure. Circulation 1996; 93: 2135-2141.

222. Bashir Y, Sneddon JF, Staunton A, et al: Effects of long-term oral magnesium chloride replacement in congestive heart failure secondary to coronary artery disease. Am J Cardiol 1993; 72: 1156-1162.

223. Packer M, Gottlieb SS, Kessler PD: Hormone-electrolyte interactions in the pathogenesis of lethal cardiac arrhythmias in patients with congestive heart failure. Am J Med 1986; 80 (Suppl 4A): 23-29

224. Schmidt U, Kuhn U, et al: Efficacy of the hawthorn (Crateagus) preparation LI 132 in 78 patients with chronic congestive heart failure defined as NYHA functional class II. Phytomed 1994; 1: 17-24.

225. Maevers VW, Hensel H: Changes in local myocardial blood flow following oral administration of a Crataegus extract to non-anesthetized dogs. Arzneim Forsch - Drug Res 1974; 24: 783-785.

226. Bahorun T, Trotin F, et al: Antioxidant activities of Crataegus monogyna extracts. Planta Med 1994; 60: 323–328.

227. Bordia A, Verma SK: Effect of vitamin C on platelet adhesiveness and platelet aggregation in coronary artery disease patients. Clin Cardiol 1985; 8: 552-554.

228. Chan AC: Vitamin E and arteriosclerosis. J Nutr 1998; 128: 1593-1596.

229. Weiser H, Vecchi M, Schlachter M: Stereoisomers of alpha-tocopheryl acetate. Internal J Vit Nutr Res 1986; 56: 45 - 56.

230. Diplock AT: Vitamin E. In: Fat-soluble vitamins. Lancaster, Basel: Pennsylvania Technomic Publ Co 1985; 154-224.

231. Weiser H, Vecchi M: Stereoisomers of alpha-tocopheryl acetate. II. Biopotencies of all eight stereoisomers, individually or in mixtures, as determined by rat resorption-gestation tests. Int J Vitam Nutr Res 1982; 52: 351-370.

232. Machlin LJ, Gabriel E, Brin M: Biopotency of alpha-tocopherols as determined by curative myopathy bioassay in the rat. J Nutr 1982; 112: 1437-1440.

233. Traber MG, Rudel LL, Burton GW, Hughes L, Ingold KU, Kayden HJ: Nascent VLDL from liver perfusions of cynomolgus monkeys are preferentially enriched in RRR - compared with SRR-alpha-tocopherol: studies using deuterated tocopherols. Lipid Res 1990; 31: 687-694.

234. Stamler JS, Mendelsohn ME, Amarante P, Smick D, Andon N, Davies PF, Cooke JP, Loscalzo J: N-Acetylcysteine potentiates platelet inhibition by endothelium-derived relaxing factor. Circ Res 1989 ;65: 789-795.

235. Singh RB, Wander GS, Rastogi A, Shukla PK, Mittal A, Sharma JP, Mehrotra SK, Kapoor R, Chopra RK: Randomized, double-blind placebo-controlled trial of coenzyme Q10 in patients with acute myocardial infarction. Cardiovasc Drugs Ther 1998; 12: 347–353.

236. http://www4.dr-rath-foundation.org/The_Hague/complaint/complaint03. htm#top

237. Nelson MR, Liew D, Bertram M, Vos T: Epidemiological modelling of routine use of low dose aspirin for the primary prevention of coronary heart disease and stroke in those aged ≥70. BMJ 2005; 330:1306.

238. Schernhammer ES, Kang JH, Chan AT, Michaud DS, Skinner HG, Giovannucci E, Colditz GA, Fuchs CS: A prospective study of aspirin use and the risk of pancreatic cancer in women. J Natl Cancer Inst 2004; 96: 22-28.

239. Jandak J, Steiner M, Richardson PD: Reduction of platelet adhesiveness by vitamin E supplementation in human. Throb Res 1988; 49: 393-404.

240. Jandak J, Steiner M, Richardson PD: α-Tocopherol, an effective inhibitor of platelet adhesion. Blood 1989; 73: 141-149.

241. Cooke JP, Tsao PS: Arginine: A new therapy for atherosclerosis? Circulation 1997; 95: 311-312.

242. Rath M: Wir suchen Architekten für ein neues Gesundheitswesen. Almelo: Matthias Rath B.V. 1998.

243. http://www4.dr-rath-foundation.org/pharmaceutical_business/laws_of_the_ pharmaceutical_industry.htm

244. http://www.pharmexec.com/pharmexec/data/articlelong/pharmexec/182002/ 17966/article.pdf

245. New York: Fortune Magazine, June 23, 1997.

246. Rath M: The Chemnitz Program. Almelo: MR Publishing.

247. Pfeiffer CC: Nutrition and mental illness. An orthomolecular approach to balancing body chemistry. Rochester: Healing Arts Press 1987.